In the Key of Genius

Adam Ockelford was born in Nottingham in 1959, grew up on the Isle of Wight, and, when he left school, studied at the Royal Academy of Music in London. It was at this time, in the late 1970s, that he first started working with blind children, including those with additional disabilities. He was fascinated by just how musical many of them seemed to be. Trying to understand how these young people could 'hear' and understand music so effectively led him to develop a theory of how music makes sense – not just to them, but to all of us – a theory for which he was awarded a PhD by London University in 1993, and that has since been published in a number of academic journals and books.

But Adam believes that theories are of little value unless they're put into practice, and he continues to work with a number of the young people – now adults – whom he first started to teach over twenty years ago, including Derek.

Adam is Professor of Music at Roehampton University; Secretary of the Society for Education, Music and Psychology Research; Chair of 'Soundabout', an Oxford-based charity that supports music provision for children with complex needs; and founder of The AMBER Trust, which provides bursaries for blind and partially sighted children to have music lessons.

D0109522

ADAM OCKELFORD

IN THE KEY OF GENIUS

OF GENIUS

The Extraordinary Life of Derek Paravicini

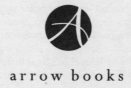

arrow books

Published by Arrow 2008

2 4 6 8 10 9 7 5 3 1

Copyright © Adam Ockelford 2007

Adam Ockelford has asserted his right under the Copyright, Designs
and Patents Act 1988 to be identified as the author of this work

This book is sold subject to the condition that it shall not,
by way of trade or otherwise, be lent, resold, hired out, or
otherwise circulated without the publisher's prior consent in any
form of binding or cover other than that in which it is published
and without a similar condition, including this condition, being
imposed on the subsequent purchaser

First published in Great Britain in 2007 by
Hutchinson
Random House, 20 Vauxhall Bridge Road,
London SW1V 2SA

www.rbooks.co.uk

Addresses for companies within The Random House Group Limited
can be found at:
www.randomhouse.co.uk/offices.htm

The Random House Group Limited Reg. No. 954009

A CIP catalogue record for this book
is available from the British Library

ISBN 9780099513582

The Random House Group Limited supports The Forest Stewardship
Council (FSC), the leading international forest certification organisation.
All our titles that are printed on Greenpeace approved FSC certified
paper carry the FSC logo. Our paper procurement policy can be found
at www.rbooks.co.uk/environment

Printed and bound in Great Britain by
CPI Bookmarque, Croydon CR0 4TD

Affectionately dedicated to
Winifred Daly
('Nanny')
1914–1997

CENTRAL ARKANSAS LIBRARY SYSTEM
ADOLPHINE FLETCHER TERRY BRANCH
LITTLE ROCK, ARKANSAS

Contents

Opening Notes

I glanced again at the diminutive figure on my right, shock of blond hair weaving incessantly from side to side with the rhythmic rocking of his head; fingers pressed so hard into his eye sockets that the globes bulged outwards from behind their lids; thumbs stuffed comfortingly (yet somehow disturbingly) deep into his mouth. He looked strangely unfamiliar in a loose white silk shirt (specially bought for the occasion), cummerbund held up with hidden safety pins, shortened dress-suit trousers and small patent leather shoes. Not for the first time that day, the whole idea of what was about to happen seemed utterly ridiculous – crazy that so much should rest on the whim of this unpredictable boy, whose weird antics usually seemed so diverting, charming even, but which now seemed only to be courting disaster. What would happen if he refused to play? Or played the wrong piece? Or, perhaps most bizarre of all, chose to play in a different key from the one the orchestra was expecting? What would happen if he just kept playing and wouldn't stop?

I tried to quell the feeling of panic rising within me ... yet in truth Derek was capable of all these things and worse. Again, I could hear Lina's words ringing in my ears: who was I to expose him to possible humiliation on such a spectacular scale? And all this without his consent (for Derek could have had no idea of what agreeing to take part would entail). Who was I to put him on such a public pedestal from which he could so easily fall? Contemplating Derek once more, engrossed in his inner world, I was at least clear about one thing: the only person feeling the pressure at that moment was *me*. Derek was blissfully unaware that the world's media had been closing in on him over the past few days and were about to subject his efforts to the closest scrutiny.

'Nanny,' said Derek, as elliptically as ever, being still for a moment.

'Yes, Nanny's sitting in the audience, waiting to hear you play,' I batted back, unthinkingly decoding what he meant, concentrating on making my voice sound a good deal calmer than I felt. I didn't want him to pick up on my nerves – but he was excited all right, and I knew it.

'You will play very well.'

I was, of course, familiar with Derek's eccentric use of pronouns.

'I hope you do, Derek – everyone will be listening! They're really looking forward to it.'

A pause, and then: '"Call me Irresponsible".'

'Yes, "Call me Irresponsible" first, then "L-O-V-E" – with the orchestra.'

We were interrupted by a knock on the door.

'This is it,' I thought, and then aloud, 'Come in!'

But it was a stranger – yet another stranger with a camera – just like the many strangers who'd been assailing us all day. I'd thought that our dressing room was off limits.

'One more photo?'

Despite my irritation at this invasion of our privacy at a time when I just *had* to keep Derek calm, there was something in the man's tone that was friendly, persuasive, not threatening, just doing his job.

'OK, OK, quick then.'

'Playing the piano?'

There was a small upright in the dressing room, but this was the last thing I wanted, with Derek primed and ready to go with his first piece. If he played 'Call me Irresponsible' now, then the Philharmonia might get more (or less) than they had bargained for when Derek got on stage.

But the photographer was already ushering us into position, somehow mindful of the fact that Derek couldn't see.

Easier to go with the flow . . . couldn't risk making a scene now.

'How about "The Entertainer", Derek, like George Shearing?' I said, quietly wresting back the initiative.

Without even seeming to check where the first notes were, Derek was off: fluently, cheekily in a jaunty up-tempo version of the Joplin number that owed little to the Shearing legacy. His fingers, so childishly contorted only minutes before, miraculously unfurled and began darting irrepressibly up and down the keyboard, as much in the air as on the notes, leaping over wide intervals with uncanny accuracy. Then, without warning, there were new chords, a jazzy rhythm; belatedly, Shearing had arrived. But no sooner had the master made his presence felt than Derek shoved him irreverently off the keyboard – *his* keyboard – with cascades of brilliant, shimmering scales, his fingers consuming the notes beneath them with an insatiable appetite for sound.

The photographer, seasoned from capturing a thousand of life's oddities and extremes, shook his head. 'How old d'you say he was?'

'Nine.'

He listened for a couple of moments more, then a shrug of the shoulders, a couple of clicks, and he was done. Very efficient. A nod to me and a hand on Derek's shoulder.

'Good luck,' and he was gone as quickly as he had arrived.

'Good luck, indeed,' I thought, wondering whether I should have been more assertive in shielding Derek from this untimely attention. I never dreamt that this one last photograph, franchised within hours to newspapers across the world, would do more than anything else to put Derek's face, his achievements and maybe even a little of his spirit in front of countless millions of people, from Liverpool to Hamburg, Cape Town to Beijing, Melbourne to Tokyo. But that was still in the future, and for now my mind was fully preoccupied with the present, not daring to think beyond the next few minutes.

I became aware that Derek had finished his version of 'The Entertainer' and had retreated into himself once more. I put my hand gently on his arm, making contact but without wishing to trespass into his inner world. Again, I reflected on the day's events. The trip to the Barbican Centre from SW19, hot and sticky from the sweltering summer heat in the car. No air-conditioning. Traffic. Noise. Fumes. Sweat trickling down my back. A heavy feeling of nausea. Radio 3 to keep Derek occupied.

At last we arrive, but nowhere to park. Driving round and round as aimlessly as my thoughts. Finally, a space, and no choice but to leave our sudorific cocoon. A short walk. Which door? Where do we have to go? Then all at once, I am leading Derek into the concert hall. He is jerking to and fro like a toy on a spring, excited without knowing why, quite beyond explanations or understanding.

'Derek!' 'Derek!' 'Over here, Derek!' From nowhere, the flashes of countless cameras. The lights bounce off Derek's face unnoticed, but he is alive to the voices. Strange voices, demanding voices, pushing, jostling. Conductor at war with the TV producer. 'Must have an interview now' . . . 'Need to rehearse' . . . 'I insist!' . . . 'I insist!' . . . 'No!' Raised voices. Another butts in. It's *News at Ten*. Derek squeezes my hand tight. I hadn't reckoned on *this*.

There's no escape until, finally, someone leads us to the sanctuary of the dressing room – 'Derek Paravacinni' scrawled on a piece of card on the door in felt pen. Spelt incorrectly as usual. George Melly's sign is on the door next to Derek's. No mistake there. (Nanny later removes both cards to keep as souvenirs.) On our own at last. Deceptive calm. A sandwich and a bottle of water arrive, but Derek is not interested in food or drink. And then the wait. I long for a walk to break the tension, but don't want to tangle with the media again.

After an eternity, Nanny arrives. Gets Derek changed. Her stubby fingers, awkward with age, struggle with the safety pins. He has to look perfect. This is *her* part in the whole enterprise, the *raison d'être* of her autumn years. My bow tie comes in for some attention too. Last goodbyes. A kiss for 'Bumpy' (as Derek is known); an unspoken expectation of me that he will come up with the goods.

Another period of heavy silence, then at last a knock on the door. It's time.

'Come on, Derek.' I take his hand.

Out into the corridor; Derek is rocking again. He can hear the orchestra now and he starts to skip along. He trips up the first step on to the stage – surely he'll fall flat on his face if he doesn't concentrate.

'Derek!' I hiss. He stills momentarily. My heart is pounding in my head. Carefully, one stair at a time, we make our way up into the wings. Suddenly the orchestra is upon us, so close that you could reach out and touch the backs of the rearmost violinists. Powerfully, professionally, perfectly, the music drives forward to its climax. What *are* we doing here? Derek listens intently. Now *his* world is there before him. Thunderous applause. Derek jumps and lets out a squeal of excitement. My head is spinning. The compère is saying something, but I can hear only a jumble of words. He looks expectantly in our direction. Derek can't wait to move.

We stumble forward together, a gawky couple. I try to appear confident, but it's difficult to see with the lights glaring and I can't think straight. I help Derek on to the piano stool, awkward in the knowledge that our every move is being followed by hundreds of pairs of curious eyes. He looks absurdly small and vulnerable sitting there, with the huge grand piano in front of him, legs dangling over the pedals. I sit down on the empty chair beside him. The conductor turns to me questioningly and raises his baton. In the audience, a subdued shuffling, murmuring and a final clearing of the throat are hastily squeezed into an expectant silence. I glance at Derek. He is visibly trembling with anticipation, twisting his fingers into knots. I look back at the conductor and nod. A silent upbeat, then the first hushed chord from the strings.

Derek's hands move inexorably towards his eyes.

Another chord sounds.

I will him to come in, but the sickening realisation dawns that he hasn't even felt to find where the keyboard is.

Derek slowly starts to rock forward.

I can't bear to look and my eyes close involuntarily.

In the darkness, time stands still.

There is nothing I can do.

For the first time in his life, he is completely on his own.

Chapter One

Fight for Survival

Mary Ann lay absolutely still, silently praying that she had been mistaken. She allowed her gaze to fall on the clock beside her hospital bed and watched intently as the second hand traced a complete circle. Nothing. She started to relax. Another minute passed – 2 a.m. exactly, she noticed. Then suddenly, without warning, the pain was back, more urgent this time, unmistakable. Mary Ann groaned aloud, as much out of despair as discomfort, and fumbled for the bell push.

She sensed that the climax to a difficult six months (and a terrible week) was near. For the last seven days, doctors had battled to prevent her going into premature labour. But now it seemed, after only twenty-six weeks, she was about to lose the twins – her second such loss in recent years. Sadness mingled with anger dissolved into fear as she heard the nurse call for help.

She felt an overwhelming sense of powerlessness amid the frantic activity that followed. Doctors, midwives and nurses appeared from nowhere, it seemed: two teams, one for each baby. There was even an anaesthetist. In a moment of troubled lucidity,

Mary Ann wondered how they had managed to assemble so quickly in the middle of the night: they must have *known* that something was about to happen. But what was the point? What *was* the point? This was 1979, and she knew all too well that no baby fourteen weeks premature had ever survived in the Royal Berks.

The pains grew in frequency and intensity. At one stage, partly hidden behind the knot of white coats, to the left-hand side of the room, Mary Ann caught sight of two incubators, standing empty. A huge, sustained contraction engulfed her. And another. Within moments, the first baby was out: a limp, pitiful scrap of humanity. Quickly, clear her airway, see if she will breathe. So it was the girl. A hazy memory stirred: girls fare better than boys. So if either baby were going to make it, this would surely be the one.

Mary Ann, her eyes still closed following the final exertion, couldn't bear to look. No one said anything, though she was aware of the frenzied drama being enacted before her. Despite herself, she listened intently. No sounds of life penetrated the controlled but increasingly desperate bustle. Not a cry. Not a murmur. Nothing. Finally, the room became quiet. Keeping her eyes shut, Mary Ann could imagine the knowing looks exchanged by the medical staff.

Too devastated to react, she sank back into a torpor. Her physical respite was short-lived, however, interrupted by the first of another series of contractions. These were weaker, though, demanding less of her than before, and the second baby was delivered with unnatural ease. This time Mary Ann knew straight away that the situation was futile and she dared to watch as a pitifully small shrimp of a child was held up – scarcely bigger than the doctor's hand. She couldn't believe just how tiny the little boy was. Floppy, lifeless. Yet perfect. Her heart ached unbearably. Gently he was laid to rest next to his sister.

'I'm so sorry.'

The doctor's eyes were kind, but clearly there was nothing he could do.

There was an awkward silence as Mary Ann struggled to frame a response. In the end she said nothing and the doctor turned slowly away, while the nurses started the miserable process of cleaning and tidying things up. No one spoke. There was nothing to say. For Mary Ann, this was the lowest point in her life. Another two children lost. Her hopes and dreams snuffed out.

But something interrupted her melancholy train of thought. Yes, there it was: the faintest of whimpers. She held her breath, aware that everyone else in the room had also stopped to listen. A pause, then there it was again: the tiniest of muffled squeaks. Now all attention turned to the two babies. And as they watched, miraculously, the boy's matchstick ribs perceptibly rose and fell.

The doctor looked back to Mary Ann, a new urgency in his eyes. 'What do you want us to do?'

Her voice, though weak, was decisive. 'Go with it,' she replied, then fell back, exhausted.

The staff, who had been putting things away in ghastly slow motion, were galvanised into action. Quickly but carefully the baby was placed in one of the incubators, which was hurriedly wheeled out of the room.

'They're taking him to the special-care unit,' a nurse informed Mary Ann. 'We'll let you know how he gets on.'

But the prognosis was poor. The hospital lacked the specialist neonatal intensive-care facilities that babies of such prematurity needed in order to survive the critical first few weeks and within the hour the hospital chaplain had christened him. Hastily, names had been chosen that reflected something of his distinguished lineage: 'Derek' after his maternal grandfather (Derek Parker-Bowles, who had died a couple of years earlier); 'Nicolas' after his father; and 'Somerset' after a paternal great-grandfather, Somerset Maugham.

It wasn't until the afternoon of the same day – 26 July – that Mary Ann was well enough to take a good look at D.N.S.P., her second son. She peered in through the clear plastic lid of the incubator. There he was, lying face down on a small blue mattress. He was dwarfed by a tiny nappy, from the bottom of which two miniature pink feet poked out, no bigger than the tips of her fingers. The nappy reached halfway up Derek's back, which was then bare to his neck. Through his thin, translucent skin, thread-like veins were visible. Tubes and wires from an alarming array of machines disappeared into bandages in his arms and up his nose. His eyes were shut, just like a newborn kitten, Mary Ann thought. She noticed a wisp of curly blond hair poking out from underneath a white woollen cap.

'Good afternoon. Sister Walker.' An assertive though kindly woman's voice cut through her pre-occupation. 'You must be Mrs Paravicini. Welcome to Buscot Ward. And what do you think of your new son?'

Mary Ann started to answer, but by now Sister Walker was in the groove: 'He's a record breaker! The smallest we've ever had – just over 700 grammes.' She smiled. 'He keeps us on our toes, don't you, Derek?' she said, glancing down at him fondly. 'Every now and then he forgets to breathe, so I have to remind him!'

Mary Ann wondered how on earth someone who was barely sentient could be reminded to breathe. The answer wasn't long in coming. Looking closely at Derek again, she became aware that his back had stopped its rhythmical rise and fall, and one of the machines began emitting a loud, continous beep.

'Derek!' exclaimed Sister Walker in a jump-lead voice that startled him back into action.

Mary Ann felt suddenly weak and muttered something about returning to bed. This knife-edge existence was more than her nerves could bear. Surely it was just a matter of time before the end came.

But it didn't. Not that day, nor the next, nor the ones that followed. Every morning, Mary Ann or Derek's father, Nic, would come for the first visit of the day to see him in the special baby unit, fully expecting to be greeted with bad news. Every morning, though, Derek was still there; and on each occasion he was a little stronger and his prospects seemed a little brighter.

One of the most touching aspects of Derek's care was his feeding regime. A small amount of milk was carefully collected from other mothers on the ward, before being mixed and refrigerated, then sent off site to be sterilised. On its return it was warmed and fed straight into Derek's stomach through a tube, since he was unable to swallow. He also received blood from Mary Ann that followed a similarly circuitous route. It took only a matter of moments to draw a small amount from her arm, which was then rushed off to a unit in Oxford for sterilisation. On its return, that same small quantity – so precious to Derek – took two hours to infuse into his arm.

The most difficult part of Derek's care, though, was monitoring his oxygen levels. This could only be done by pricking one of his fingers and removing a single drop of blood for testing. Inevitably, this painstaking, painful procedure took time, so it was impossible to prevent his 'sats' swinging up and down uncontrollably. At the time, the family were not aware of the physiological effects that these fluctuations were having, though the medical staff, of course, knew all too well. Best, they thought, not to worry Nic and Mary Ann at this stage, though, when the faint flicker of hope in their hearts was starting to take hold, despite their conscious attempts to suppress it.

In the middle of his second week, however, disaster struck when Derek contracted a chest infection. More tubes were inserted as he was ventilated to keep him alive. On three terrible occasions, the cardiac monitor went completely still as Derek's heart – only the size of a grape – gave up the unequal struggle, and each time desperate efforts were made to resuscitate him.

Against all the odds, he pulled through. As the nursing staff's own written account puts it: 'Derek was determined to be a survivor.' Their record shows that he was in hospital for a total of thirteen weeks, during which time there were increasingly more 'ups' than 'downs'. At two months he took his first sip of milk from a bottle, although the nasal feeding tube remained in place for some time afterwards. Then, on 25 October, the momentous day arrived when Derek was deemed fit to be discharged. He weighed just over two kilograms and was effectively still three weeks premature.

It was at this point, although of course Derek didn't know it, that one of the most influential people in his life moved centre stage. Derek clearly needed someone very special to look after him and, in the family's view, there was only one person for the job. Miss Winifred Daly, known to readers of the *Sunday Times* as 'Nanny Parker-Bowles', but to all her friends, acquaintances and complete strangers alike simply as 'Nanny', was summoned back from her retirement flat in the Peabody Estate, Hammersmith to the family home in Warfield, near Ascot.

At a little over five feet tall, Nanny was not someone with whom Fate would tangle lightly. She was conviction personified: Nanny didn't *think* things, she *knew* them. She was the rock of good-natured, down-to-earth assurance that Mary Ann and her brothers, Andrew, Simon and Rick, had relied on as children in the 1940s and 1950s. Now, quite un-expectedly, at the age of sixty-five, her career was given a new lease of life: the start of an Indian summer that she did not regret for one moment in the challenging years that followed, despite the many times when Derek would have caused her to scratch her head, had such a thing been decorous through her blue rinse. She was a woman of deep faith and, as far as she was concerned, Derek's survival was God's will: while He had attended spiritually to things over the past three months, it was now down to Nanny to take care of matters temporal.

She wasted no time. 'For goodness' sake, Mary Ann, you can't let him out of the hospital with only *that* on!' – pointing to his little white cardigan. 'He'll catch his death.' She reached for a blanket. Never had Nanny wrapped up a baby so tightly against the autumn chill in the air.

It was strange having Derek at home after such a long time of seeing him only in hospital. He still seemed ridiculously tiny, Mary Ann mused, on the lap of his nine-year-old sister Libbet as she was allowed to hold him briefly under Nanny's watchful gaze in the nursery. Libbet had been longing to see him and hold him and play with him, having only had tantalising glimpses of her new brother in the Polaroid photographs that had been taken in the hospital and propped up on the mantelpiece. And now here he was, asleep, his head in the crook of her arm, little pink face still screwed up like a flower bud, not yet completely unfurled. He was so irresistible that she simply couldn't take her eyes off him.

It was a few days, though, before Nanny would allow the family's three dogs, Tay the black Labrador, Nic's whippet Hattie, and Nina the old Jack Russell, to satisfy their curiosity and give the newcomer a proper sniff. Nonetheless, the trio made their presence felt, barking more vociferously than ever if anyone should approach the house or the scrunch of tyres was heard on the long gravel drive, instinctively protecting the newest and most vulnerable member of their pack. Tom, the tabby cat, seemed more vocal too, pining for his usual share of attention. It was a long time before Nanny would trust *him* to go near Derek. Whenever someone opened the side door next to the nursery, a faint smell of the stables wafted in, and there was the regular clatter of hooves in the yard from one or more of the many horses that played such a big part in life at North Lodge Farm in those days: a mixture of finely bred polo ponies, racehorses and resting army mounts, though none had more affection bestowed upon it than the children's own pony Bootsie, an ancient strawberry roan.

Nanny wondered how Derek would react to this blooming, buzzing world of rich and varied sensations after knowing only the sterile environment of the special baby care unit. Surely he would be anxious or restive, missing the safe and comfortable confines of his hospital cot? But Derek seemed to take all the fresh experiences in his stride and to be perfectly content in his new home.

Strangely content, Nanny thought as, later on that first evening, she switched off the light in his bedroom. She had made up a bed next to his cot so that she could attend to him in the night whenever she was needed. Now she viewed her new charge fondly as her eyes gradually grew accustomed to the dim light. He was already peacefully asleep, and little by little she felt able to relax.

Over the next few days, Derek's life gradually settled into a new routine: an unvarying daily pattern of sleeping, feeding, being changed and gently stimulated in what at first were three-hour cycles. Every afternoon, weather permitting, there was a short walk outside in the pram so that he could benefit from the fresh country air. Most evenings there were visitors, family and friends, all keen to see Derek and remark on what a miracle his survival had been, how small he still was and so good-natured! And how was Nanny? What was it like, starting again with a new baby at her age?

'You're only as old as you feel,' Nanny would say, somewhat stiffly, and Derek's arrival had certainly charged her with a new vitality. A glorious feeling of warmth permeated her whole being, and she felt a fresh sense of purpose and a youthful energy that she thought had deserted her years before.

Duty done, the visitors were ushered out and it was bedtime. Derek always slept well, for which Nanny was thankful, though he still seemed wholly unconcerned about the dark, which continued to puzzle her. One night, when he was obviously still awake, she deliberately switched the light back on and then off again. As ever, there was no response. Once more, on and off. Nothing.

'Mary Ann!' Despite her ever-present composure, Nanny couldn't disguise the anxiety in her voice. 'Mary Ann! I think there's something wrong with Derek's eyes.'

'Nonsense!' Mary Ann came upstairs, though, and turned the light back on so she could scrutinise her young son for herself. There he was, lying with his eyes open, contentedly looking at the ceiling, or so it seemed to her. She waved her hand in front of his face. He didn't react. She tried again, her hand closer this time. Still no reaction.

'Derek!' she said apprehensively, and at last he did respond, startling to the sudden sound of her voice.

Both women looked at each other, though neither said anything.

Eventually, Nanny turned and switched off the light. 'Come on,' she said, 'we'll phone the doctor in the morning.'

It was two long weeks before the family's worst suspicions were confirmed. Nic and Mary Ann had to take Derek to London's Moorfields Eye Hospital to be seen by a paediatric ophthalmologist. He would have to be examined under anaesthetic, a distressing prospect. But the examination didn't take long, and afterwards the consultant came straight to the point: 'I'm sorry to tell you that your child is blind.'

A stunned silence followed. Nic glanced at Mary Ann, his mind reeling. He had been hoping that Nanny and Mary Ann had somehow been mistaken.

'Can anything be done?'

'I'm afraid not.' And the doctor proceeded to give

a technical explanation of what had happened to Derek's eyes during those long days in the incubator. He had developed a condition called *retrolental fibroplasia* (today known as *retinopathy of prematurity* or 'RoP'). This had resulted from the uncontrolled levels of oxygen in his blood, which had caused certain vessels in Derek's eyes to grow abnormally. These had damaged Derek's retinas – the thin, light-sensitive films at the backs of his eyes.

Nic wanted to ask another question, but the consultant was in full flow.

Normally, the retina was made up of over a hundred million receptors called 'rods' and 'cones', which sent messages down the optic nerves to the brain. In Derek's case, however, the retinas had become detached as a result of the scarring . . .

Nic interrupted him. He had to know. 'So there really is no hope at all?'

The consultant met Nic's gaze with some difficulty. 'No. I'm sorry.' He paused briefly, then added, 'I'll register him today.'

Register him? The words hung balefully in the air. What did the doctor mean, exactly? But it was clear that their son, who had fought so hard to survive, was to be disabled for the rest of his life. It was too much to take in. Nic couldn't look at Mary Ann. Somehow, they found their way out of the room and met up with Nanny who had been waiting with Derek as he came round from the anaesthetic.

The drive home through the London rush hour seemed interminable, the gloomy silence in the car broken only by the bustle of the traffic outside.

Nanny listened intently to Mary Ann's fractured account of what had been said. Stoical as ever, she had already been planning what to do. Toys that make sounds, that's what he needs, she thought, and as Nic pulled out on to Hammersmith Broadway, she started to make a mental note of the possibilities.

That night, Nanny made another decision: since Derek couldn't see her, whenever she wasn't physically in contact with him she had better keep in touch by talking or singing. So she got into the habit of telling him everything that she was doing, what was in the room around him, what she could see out of the window, what the weather was like, and so on. And when Nanny wasn't talking, she was singing: all the nursery rhymes from her vast repertoire, songs from the shows insofar as she could remember them, and popular songs from her youth. At first, of course, Derek didn't know what any of this meant, but he quickly got used to Nanny's voice – a constant mellow stream in a complex and ever-changing auditory landscape – and by the time he was three he could do a creditable impression of her 'warbling'.

Intuitively, Nanny intensified the daily routine, helping Derek to anticipate what was coming next by letting him smell his clean clothes before dressing him, for example, and always remembering to tap her fingers on the bottle before feeding time. Over the weeks and months that followed, Derek grew accustomed to these and a range of other household sounds too: the radio in the utility room that Alice, the daily, liked to have on while she did the ironing; the television in the drawing room; and, in time,

Derek's own 'noisy toys'. Nanny had bought just about every conceivable sound-making toy for him, though Derek didn't seem to play with these at all in the conventional sense, she noticed. He wasn't interested in exploring what she gave him in any systematic way or testing it to see what it could do. Derek would simply bang whatever was handed to him on anything that was available: the tray on his high chair, the floor or another toy. He would keep going relentlessly until even Nanny's patience was exhausted.

Derek's fingers, though still tiny, were extraordinary too. They were constantly on the move, curling and uncurling and twisting over themselves like the tentacles of a baby octopus. His hands also developed some habits that made less comfortable viewing. Sometimes, clenching his fists, he would push them hard into his closed eyes. On other occasions he would put both thumbs in his mouth and extend his forefingers upwards, poking at his eyelids. Strangely, these behaviours seemed to cause Derek no distress, and if anyone gently tried to lower his hands from his face they invariably found their way straight back up again. At the same time, when he was lying down, Derek's head would weave relentlessly from side to side. And later, once he could sit up, he would rock to and fro as well.

Why does he do this? Nanny wondered. In all her years of bringing up children she had never seen behaviour like it. Perhaps it was usual for blind babies? After all, he couldn't see what he was doing (or what anyone else did, for that matter). Or perhaps there was more to it than that – but this was a line of thought that she couldn't bear to contemplate, so instead she picked up her 'Blessing' (as she referred to Derek) and gave him an enormous hug. He giggled with pleasure. For above all, despite his penchant for self-stimulation, he loved human company: to be in contact with other people through their touch or sound or scent (later, as a child, he would identify people first by smelling their hands). He relished being held and tickled, and bounced up and down. And he delighted in hearing familiar voices, which for him signalled the presence of family or friends, many of whom were to remain loyal companions throughout his childhood and beyond.

At first, having heard that Derek was blind, those who had previously dropped in to see him without giving it a second thought now approached the nursery with some awkwardness – trepidation even – but no one could feel sad or sorry for Derek for long: from his earliest days at North Lodge Farm he seemed to exude a natural charm that people found captivating.

A favourite visitor was 'Godfather Patrick' (Lord Patrick Beresford) who shared the family's love of horses, having been one of England's highest-ranked polo players, winning the prestigious Cowdray Gold Cup twice. Not that any of this was remotely important to baby Derek, who just loved his godfather's infectious laugh. Patrick had the marvellous quality of somehow being able to convey in his voice the mischievous twinkle that others could see in his eye, and he struck up an immediate rapport with his godson. He would often drop in on Sunday evenings just as Nanny turned on the television for *Songs of Praise*. As Patrick remarked, Derek seemed to find the sound of the hymns particularly attractive, and he would listen intently to the singing and the sound of the organ, fingers pressed in his eyes but his head, for once, quite still.

Patrick was one of a group of close family friends and relatives who were well aware of the reason why Derek had lost his sight, and Nic and Mary Ann were astonished when, quite unsolicited, donations started to arrive discreetly at North Lodge Farm. These were intended to enable the Royal Berks to purchase the latest neonatal intensive-care equipment so that premature babies in the future could benefit from the new technology that had not been available for Derek. In particular, it was vital that the hospital obtained one of the new transcutaneous oxygen monitors so that they could take continuous readings and avoid the uncontrolled fluctuations that had damaged Derek's eyes. Unobtrusively, over £37,000 was raised in just a few weeks: as Mary Ann said to Nanny, the first tangible good that had come out of Derek's misfortune. She could never in her wildest dreams have imagined the extent of the good that was yet to come.

It hardly seemed any time at all before Derek's first year had passed and his birthday was due – albeit three and half months before it should have been. It seemed incredible now that he should have been a November baby. The day, 26 July, dawned grey but fine, and Nanny was up particularly early to make sure that all was prepared and perfect for the afternoon's party. Amid the balloons and the jelly and the birthday cake, Derek gurgled happily, absorbing the sounds of excitement around him and banging the tray on his high chair with his spoon. Nanny was attentive as ever, ensuring everyone ate their fill and leading the singing of 'Happy Birthday'. Libbet helped Derek to blow out the solitary candle. Charles, his brother, assisted in cutting the cake. Nic and Mary Ann chatted convivially with their guests.

But deep down, although they hadn't yet confided in each other, the three adults were increasingly wondering what the future might hold for Derek. He seemed to be rocking more and more these days, and his fingers rarely left his eyes. There were strange depths to the young boy that they couldn't fathom. Whenever he was left alone he appeared to retreat into an inner world whose nature they could only guess. At these times Nanny yearned to see behind those sightless eyes and into Derek's mind to find out what he was thinking. Unbeknown to her, the clues were already there, but it would be some time yet before she understood the extraordinary developmental route that Derek was charting for himself.

Chapter Two

Kitten on the Keys

Nanny paused halfway across the bridge and lifted Derek out of his pram, allowing the breeze to play with his newly grown curls of blond hair. She gently smoothed them down. 'Just like your father's,' she said, partly to herself. Derek's face was radiant in the early evening sunshine, his cheeks flushed from his day by the sea. He was no longer startled by the screech of herring gulls wheeling overhead and now, from below, he was intrigued by the irregular rhythm of the waves lapping on the ancient stone piers of the Longbridge.

Nanny had left the rest of the family refreshing themselves in Bideford, the north Devonshire town where they had taken a holiday cottage, and had gone off with Derek for a walk by the quay and on over the River Torridge. As she looked about her for something of interest to describe to him, the characteristic white superstructure of the MS *Oldenberg* came into view as the old German ferry rounded a bend in the distance. She was plying her way slowly upriver with a gaggle of day trippers returning from a birdwatching trip to Lundy Island.

'The big ship sails on the alley alley oh,' Nanny began, without thinking, rocking Derek back and forth as she sang. He giggled with pleasure. Inwardly, Nanny smiled too: she loved these intimate moments with him, when his experience of the world was mediated by her alone and he was not distracted by other voices, other personalities, jostling for his attention.

As the *Oldenberg* drew closer, the low throb of her engine gradually grew perceptible, then physically palpable in the air, and Derek became quite still in Nanny's arms as he gave this new sound, this novel sensation, his full attention. She had noticed this about him before: whereas other one-year-olds would instinctively turn towards the source of a sound to see what was making it, Derek often appeared not to react at all. At first, Nanny had been alarmed by his apparent lack of response (was there something wrong with his ears too?), but she soon realised that Derek was actually able to attend to sounds best by keeping completely still, head down.

Sensing his focus on the deep grumbling of the engine, she felt the urge, as always, to tell him what it was. 'That's a ship', she said, 'that's come all the way from Lundy Island.'

As ever, Derek loved to hear her voice, though with no visual hooks to hang Nanny's words on they came across as just another stream of sound. For although no one realised it at the time, while the parts of his brain that processed what he heard were becoming more and more refined, they were not getting linked up in the usual way with the parts that dealt with concepts and their representation as words. So for him, the deep throbbing in the air and Nanny saying the word 'ship' were both equally valid grist to his auditory mill, but the two were not meaningfully connected.

The highly eccentric manner in which Derek's brain was wiring itself up was to have a profound effect on him in future years, eventually giving rise to one of the most extraordinary minds of our time, unique in its particular cocktail of extreme abilities and inabilities. But for now, just like other babies, Derek intuitively craved new experiences that would fuel his development. He had been blissfully happy feeling the sand and the sea swirling round his toes as Mary Ann held him at the water's edge. He loved the drive home in the car with the family chatting, arguing and laughing all around him, music from the radio playing and the wind swishing in from Nic's partly open window. And when they got back to North Lodge Farm, he laughed aloud as he was jolted this way and that by the ambling gait of Bootsie, Nanny's familiar voice at his side warning Libbet to take care as she led the children's pony.

So August passed, summer turned to early autumn, and Charles and Libbet, who had spent so much of their time cuddling, cajoling, teasing and tickling their little brother, returned to school. The days at North Lodge Farm became quieter again, and Nanny was worried that Derek seemed to be missing their lively interaction and was retreating into himself once more. Left to his own devices, he would rock and poke his eyes ever more obsessively (surely he would damage them if he went on like that?) and the wear and tear on his toys grew worse as they were clattered together with increasing strength and precision. At least they could be replaced, Nanny thought, but she was uncomfortable with the fact that Derek seemed wholly unable to engage with anything purposefully unless someone was there to encourage him. As soon as he was left alone, his strange behaviour would start up again.

What could she find that would interest him, that would draw him out of himself, that would make him want to explore the world productively on *his* terms? Whatever it was would have to entail making sounds, for sure, but it couldn't involve anything that Derek could pick up and bang, since that would just set off one of his repetitive cycles of behaviour that led nowhere.

Nanny looked around the kitchen, where she was preparing Derek's tea, and her eyes lighted on the everyday objects that had kept Charles and Libbet and countless generations of other children happy for hours: pots and pans, a large wooden spoon, the egg whisk and several drawers of cutlery. Perhaps not!

Then her glance fell on a Parker-Bowles family photo and a memory began to stir. Maybe there *was* something that would do the trick. He was far too young for it, of course, but what she had in mind had long been superseded, so no one would be upset if Derek treated it roughly. Was it still around, though? There was only one way to find out. Moving the pan whose contents she had absent-mindedly been stirring off the Aga's hotplate, Nanny called to Ester, a Filipino maid who was also very much part of the family, to help her up into the loft.

With some difficulty, Nanny pushed aside skiing paraphernalia, old hatboxes, a croquet set, a crate with books in . . . and then she saw it, partly hidden behind an old suitcase. She untangled the lead from a standard lamp and pulled it into view. There it was: Derek Parker-Bowles's small electric organ that he had bought some years ago from Woolworths – she couldn't now remember exactly when or why. Nanny blew the dust off the keys. One note was a little out of line, but otherwise its two and a half octaves or so seemed to be in order. With Ester's help, she took the instrument downstairs into the nursery, wiped it over with a cloth and somewhat cautiously plugged it in. But she needn't have worried: the familiar whirring started up just as it had always done. Nanny tried the notes one at a time. A couple didn't make a sound, and another tended to stick down, but all in all she was pleased with her find. How would Derek react?

She didn't have to wait long to find out. The unfamiliar tones had roused him from his afternoon nap and, curious to see what would happen, Nanny sat him straight down on the floor in front of the keyboard. She started to play a few notes, but was overwhelmed by the immediacy and intensity of Derek's response. He emitted a shriek of delight and leant forward, both hands reaching out, urgently trying to locate the source of this new, bewitching sound. With his palms he pushed down several keys at a time, producing a cacophony that animated him even more. He started slapping the notes, then, beside himself with excitement, thumped them with such ferocity that the whole keyboard shook.

'Derek!' said Nanny, at once amazed and perturbed, and unsure what to do.

He didn't hear her. Reaching up above his head, he brought both his small fists down with astonishing rapidity and force. A knot of sounds spluttered from the organ. Again his hands went up . . .

But Nanny had had enough and was already standing up to turn the organ off. So when Derek hit the keys again, nothing happened. For a moment he scrabbled at them desperately. But the sound wouldn't come back. He cried out, clutching at the keyboard in anguish. Still no sound. Then there was a pause while he took a breath.

Although Nanny knew what was coming, even she was taken aback by the strength of the eruption that followed: a fervid outpouring of sorrow, frustration and rage. His face bright red, Derek screamed and screamed. He lashed out, kicking and thumping.

This was *not* the kind of behaviour that Nanny would tolerate from anyone – not even Derek – and she rapidly decided that a change of scene was called for. Without a word, she whisked him up and into his pushchair, strapped him in securely and set off for a walk. How long they were out would depend on Derek, though in Nanny's experience the mixture of fresh air and the calming motion of the buggy quickly quietened young children. But Derek was very agitated, and they had to go the entire length of the drive and halfway round the lake at the side of North Lodge Farm before his equilibrium was restored.

Then Nanny had time to reflect. Of course, she'd seen countless of her young charges get overexcited and witnessed more temper tantrums than she cared to remember, but the sheer passion of Derek's reaction to the organ and then to it being removed astonished her. She smiled to herself and shook her head. She'd certainly succeeded in finding something that Derek wanted to do on his own! But how could she get him to play constructively with his new find without destroying it?

As it happened, Derek was out all the next day at a hospital appointment – he still had to go for regular check-ups – and then, being half-term, Nanny had arranged to take him away to visit her great friend and fellow nanny, Dom, in the north. So it was a little while before Derek got to try out the organ again. Then one day, after lunch, when he tended to be at his calmest, Nanny sat him down in front of the organ again and, with some trepidation, turned it on. This time the whirring sound alone was enough to tell Derek what was there and as before he leant forward and attacked the keys eagerly. To her relief, Nanny judged that he was exploring the notes more carefully this time, although again it wasn't long before the fists started.

'No, Derek!' she said firmly and turned the organ off. And then in a quieter voice, 'Gently!'

He paused. She turned it back on.

Derek started to investigate the keyboard again in

a more measured way, before gradually getting more excited.

'Derek!'

This time Nanny didn't have to resort to the power switch.

And so the routine was established and another link in this most curious of symbiotic relationships was forged. Nanny had found a way of keeping Derek occupied and exerting some control over him using only her voice, and although he wasn't consciously aware of it, Derek had found a way of controlling Nanny just by making different sounds.

Of course, Derek couldn't spend his entire time playing around with the organ (Nanny decided) and she continued her search for other activities that would interest him. Now, at eighteen months, he was at least crawling around the nursery and, best of all, he loved crashing around in his baby-walker: indeed, he seemed to enjoy deliberately colliding with things, particularly Nanny's legs as she worked in the kitchen.

'Bumpity bump!' exclaimed Nanny as the walker caught her on the back of the knee.

Derek giggled with pleasure.

He wheeled himself away from her in preparation for another attack, but instead ricocheted off his high chair and straight into the leg of the kitchen table.

'Bump, bump, bump!' Nanny laughed. 'We shall have to call you Bumpy, won't we?' And then, without thinking, 'Come on, Bumps, it's time for lunch.'

The nickname was so apt that it caught on with

family and friends immediately, and has prevailed ever since. 'Derek' is reserved for public occasions and serious misdemeanours!

It was Libbet who first noticed the change. The Easter holidays were drawing to a close and she had spent most of the previous two weeks with her Bumpy in the nursery, playing rough-and-tumble games, digging through his toy box to find things he hadn't come across recently, reading him stories, and rocking him to and fro on the family's child-sized wooden rhino. It was now Friday afternoon and, worn out by his boundless energy, she lay on the floor and left him to play alone with the little organ for a while. She was so accustomed to the complex blur of sounds that her brother somehow managed to get the thing to produce, that she didn't notice anything different to begin with. But she gradually became aware that the sounds that were emanating from the organ were actually quite melodious: nothing she could recognise as being particularly this tune or that; more like a church organist marking time before the service started. She sat up to get a better view of what he was doing. Initially, he seemed to be deploying his usual jumble of fists and palms and knuckles, but it gradually dawned on her that his hands were in reality moving together, systematically up and down the keys, black and white. Without disturbing him, she leant over to watch more closely. Despite his erratic hand movements, he was somehow consistently managing to play two notes with the right hand and two with the left, with more or less regular spaces between them.

'Quick!' cried Libbet excitedly to Nanny who was in the utility room finishing off some ironing. 'Come and listen. Bumpy's playing some music.'

Dubiously but dutifully, Nanny put down the iron and came in to the nursery to find out what was happening.

Peering over Libbet's shoulder, she too could see the pattern of the notes that Derek was pressing down, though it didn't sound like a recognisable piece to her. Still, it was a vast improvement on the thumping of three months earlier and, come to think of it, by far the cleverest thing that he had ever managed to do. She suddenly felt very proud.

'That's *lovely*, Bumps,' she said. Derek Parker-Bowles would have approved, she was sure.

Little did Nanny and Libbet realise, though, that this was just the first outward sign of the extraordinary developments that we now know must have been going on in Derek's brain. His fascination with abstract patterns of sound, those thousands of hours spent simply *listening* during the first twenty months of his life, largely uncontaminated by understanding, had caused millions of special neuronal connections to form, and it was those connections that now lay behind the emergence of a precocious musicality. What Libbet and Nanny had witnessed was rather like the first glimpse of a beautiful butterfly emerging from a chrysalis – though, of course, they had no idea that they had only seen the tip of one wing and that there was much more to come.

As far as Derek was concerned, each musical note was coming to have a distinct personality: familiar friends in a confusing world. So when he heard a choir sing or an orchestra play, he was developing the ability to tell exactly which note each singer or instrumentalist was producing. Being given the organ to play had opened up a whole new realm of possibilities. One day, by chance, he must have allowed his fingers to unfurl enough to play individual notes, one at a time or in the patterns needed to make recognisable chords. Something must have 'clicked' in his brain: Derek's own 'eureka moment'. No one knows exactly when or how long the realisation took to dawn. But what Derek had stumbled on was the fact that the music that he had heard 'out there' – or at least parts of it – he could now reproduce for himself, rather like the babbling that usually precedes a baby's first recognisable words.

The chords that Libbet and Nanny observed were the first discernible evidence of that process in action. Derek was able to recreate some of the building blocks of music, but he hadn't yet acquired the skills to put them together to form whole melodies.

Again, it was Libbet who noticed the next stage in Derek's development, some months later. It was a wet Sunday afternoon in September. Nic and Mary Ann were in the drawing room, relaxing after lunch. Libbet burst in. 'Quick, quick, come and see, Derek's playing that hymn we sang in church!'

They didn't believe her, of course. And by the time they had been persuaded to join her in the nursery, Derek had reverted to his 'organist warming up' routine, hands tracing their familiar parallel paths up and down the keyboard.

'Play the hymn, Derek, play the hymn!' Libbet urged him.

Derek didn't understand, but, pleased to have her company and realising that she was within reach, gleefully stretched out his right hand to muss her hair. His left, meantime, continued its measured steps up the keys, as though wholly unaware of what the other one was up to.

'Derek, stop messing about and play the hymn,' Libbet remonstrated, removing his hand from her head and placing it back on the keyboard.

Sensing a fight in prospect, Derek laughed and went to grab her hair with both hands.

Tearfully, Libbet caught hold of his wrists. 'Derek, play the hymn, play the hymn!'

But Nic had already given Mary Ann a knowing look and was returning to his newspaper in the drawing room. She followed him with a sigh. They were both delighted that Derek and his sister got on so well, but she'd obviously imagined that he'd been playing real music – the idea was just too preposterous to contemplate.

Libbet, meanwhile, stung by the combination of their disbelief and Derek's lack of co-operation – especially with *her* – was too upset to mention his playing again. As it turned out, though, her vindication was not long in coming.

It was the middle of the following week and Nanny was sitting in the nursery, keeping an eye on Derek while she sorted out a photograph album. She had always been meticulous in keeping the family's pictorial record of events in order and Derek's arrival had provided her with a wealth of fresh material. Each photograph was carefully chosen (more for its content than the quality of the image) before being fixed into the album, dated and labelled. 'There!' she said to herself, completing the page on their recent holiday in Southport. She sat back to admire her efforts and the memories came flooding back. A glorious summer's day. Derek losing the unequal battle with his first ice cream. Libbet building sand-castles for him to knock over with his blue plastic spade. A huge expanse of sandy beach, with the Irish Sea in the distance. Nanny's eyes were closed now. She could feel the warm sun on her back, smell the fronds of drying seaweed and hear the children's voices, laughing and shouting. The strains of 'Molly Malone' were coming from somewhere. It was one of her favourites. She had often sung it for Derek, and before she knew it she found herself joining in: 'She was a fishmonger, and sure 'twas no wonder, for so were . . .'

She awoke with a jolt, with the music still ringing in her ears. She blinked and looked around. Derek was still there, bashing about on his keyboard as ever. It must have been his playing that had made her think of 'Molly Malone'. She focused on him fondly for a moment and became aware that he wasn't playing his usual chords. He seemed to be producing a new concoction of sounds she hadn't heard him come up with before, though the overall effect sounded strangely familiar. And then, as she watched, she realised what it was: before her very eyes he distinctly picked out the chorus of the old

Irish folksong using the side of the little finger on his right hand in a series of deliberate chopping movements. His left hand seemed to be producing some sort of accompaniment. She must still be dreaming, she decided, shaking her head, though any thought of trying to wake herself up was overcome by the irresistible urge to join in. 'Alive, alive oh! Alive, alive oh!' she sang, and Derek carried on, following her now, his head weaving vigorously from side to side, his body rocking to and fro, his whole being transported by the music they were making. 'Crying cockles, and mussels, alive, alive oh!' Voice and keyboard ended together, triumphantly.

For the first time in her life, Nanny was completely at a loss for words. There was even a tear in her eye. She gave Derek the most enormous hug. He was pleased, though perplexed by the strength of her sudden attention and, freeing himself, started to play again.

'Mary Ann. *Mary Ann!* Come and listen to this. You won't believe your ears.'

Mary Ann was used to the hyperbole that invariably greeted each of Derek's new achievements: finally managing to sit up in the bath, being able to say 'dada' (repeatedly) and at last taking a step on his own by holding on to the furniture. What was it this time? She could hear from Nanny's tone that non-attendance was not an option, though, and with curiosity banishing any of the reluctance that she might have felt, she made her way up the steps from the kitchen and put her head round the nursery door.

Nanny started singing again and Derek joined in on the keyboard, with a more elaborate accompaniment this time, using both hands as before. All three verses. There was no doubting it: he really could play. And with such feeling!

Mary Ann could only smile at Nanny in disbelief. Her son truly was amazing. How could it be that this little boy, just over two years old, totally blind, virtually unable to speak and apparently able to understand very little of what was going on in the world, had taught himself to play the keyboard – something that she couldn't even do herself? It just didn't seem possible, yet she had seen and heard it happen.

Derek's miraculous new achievement was the main attraction at North Lodge Farm for the next few weeks: he enjoyed being the centre of attention and he was happy to perform his party trick for anyone who cared to listen (and everyone invariably did). Lord Patrick in particular was thrilled at his godson's unlikely accomplishment and applauded heartily each time the piece came to an end. For Derek, this applause was the most tangible expression of the excitement he could sense in those around him and he grew to love – indeed, to expect – clapping at the conclusion of every performance. As a result, the sad tale of Molly Malone tended to get shorter and shorter! As soon as he had taken his hands off the keys, Derek would join in his own ovation with as much relish and energy as he had just put into his playing.

Other pieces soon followed. There were children's

songs, such as 'I Can Sing a Rainbow', Nanny's favourites, including 'In an English Country Garden', and hits like Shakin' Stevens's 'Green Door'. Just how much Derek was listening to things and taking them in without anyone realising was tellingly brought home one day when he started playing the theme tune from the television series *The Flame Trees of Thika*. As the episodes weren't aired until well after Nanny had put Derek to bed (and, she had always assumed, he was sound asleep), questions were asked in the house, much to her chagrin and everyone else's amusement! What else might he have heard and remembered, the family wondered. There was no way of knowing: everything except music remained firmly locked in Derek's head and even this could be hard to retrieve. Unless you could sing him the beginning of a piece or knew precisely the name he associated with it, there was no way of conveying what you meant (as Libbet had discovered to her cost with the incident of the hymn).

It was becoming obvious that Derek was fast outgrowing his grandfather's little plastic keyboard and Nic suggested letting him try his Yamaha organ that until now had unobtrusively occupied one corner of the drawing room. Its polished wooden case housed two manuals, each with forty-four notes, and it had an integral pedal board that spanned a complete octave. Surrounding the pair of keyboards was an impressive array of different coloured knobs, buttons and sliders. By virtue of the latest electronic wizardry, these could variously create a range of different sounds (though they were all unmistakably 'Yamaha'), activate popular dance rhythms and introduce special effects, including vibrato. This last control was the one that particularly interested Derek, ever since his brother Charles, sitting next to him on the organ's bench, had discovered that it made the sounds wobble rather like Nanny's singing. On hearing the effect, everyone had started warbling like a choir of dissipated opera singers, quickly collapsing into uncontrollable fits of laughter – Derek included.

Nanny, as ever, had taken it in good part. She was quietly thrilled at Derek's delight as he explored his new universe of sounds. He charted the unfamiliar territory, she noticed, by repeatedly feeling up and down until he reached the notes at the top and bottom extremes of the lower manual, which was all he could easily reach at first. He beamed with pleasure at his new-found freedom – those twelve extra keys – though from time to time he still loved to return to his grandfather's keyboard, his first musical voice.

Nic, too, was delighted when one day Derek quite spontaneously crawled over to him and clambered up on to his knee as he sat at the organ, where he had been painstakingly working out the tune and accompaniment for 'Don't Cry for Me, Argentina' from a book of special Yamaha arrangements. With Lilliputian hands, less than a quarter the size of his father's, Derek instinctively reached out and showed him how the song should sound. Nic was humbled, amused, astonished. His son exuded a simple, joyous musicality that he had never experienced before. Derek didn't need dots on a piece of paper or colour-coded buttons to tell him what to do. For him, it seemed, making music was the most natural thing in the world.

With half an eye on the future, Nanny decided that Derek's burgeoning talents should be challenged through exposure to a more 'serious' repertoire: after all, if he could learn TV theme tunes by ear, then presumably he could do the same with classical music? It really would be something if he could learn some *Beethoven*, for example. That would put the extent of his musical abilities beyond question.

Of course, such values were foreign to Derek: what made 'Green Door' 'music' was essentially the same as what made a Beethoven symphony 'music'. Both were constructed from the same basic building blocks of sound and it was only the surface detail, particularly the instruments that were used, that made them different and meant that one should be assigned to the 'classical' category while the other was designated as 'rock'. But Derek's eclectic musical mind didn't respect boundaries like these. As far as he was concerned, music did not fall into two categories: 'serious' and 'fun'. For him, with no awareness of social norms or prejudices, all music was *serious fun*, all of it of equal merit, all of it worthy of the same meticulous attention.

Nanny entered the music shop with some trepidation. She was back up in Hammersmith for a couple of days, having a break from the Paravicini household. Ester would have to look after Derek on her own. Now, how would she go about choosing a record? There were hundreds in the 'classical' section. In the end Nanny followed the assistant's suggestion and went for the latest recording by the up-and-coming Richard Clayderman – the height of serious piano playing, she was assured, and he was *so* good-looking, with blond hair, just like her Bumps.

As it turned out, Nanny couldn't have made a better choice. The aspiring Prince of the Drawing-Room Organ got on famously with piano's King of Kitsch. Clayderman's idiosyncratic habit of 'improving' on the great composers by adding extra chords and runs suited Derek down to the ground. Of course, he could never have explained in words why he felt such an affinity with Clayderman's way of playing. But it seems likely that it was the Frenchman's naturally free-and-easy style of performance, in which *self*-expression was the order of the day rather than any thought of fidelity to the composer's intentions, that accorded so strongly with Derek's own developing musical instincts. So the Clayderman influence was irresistible and more pieces rapidly became established in Derek's repertoire: Beethoven's 'Für Elise', Schubert's 'Ave Maria', the 'Raindrop' Prelude by Chopin and 'The Swan' from Saint-Saëns's *Carnival of the Animals*.

Just how Derek did it continued to perplex those around him. He didn't seem to practise one hand then the other before trying them both together in the usual way. He didn't divide pieces up into manageable chunks, initially attempting the opening bars, for example, and working away at those, before moving on to the next section, then the one after that and so on. In fact, Derek didn't seem to *practise* at all. He played a good deal, that was for sure, usually for several hours a day (although Nanny tried to limit him to three – otherwise, she feared, he never *would* learn to do anything else). And as he played, new pieces just came tumbling out of him, all at once.

His first efforts, particularly of longer or more complicated works, were often like sketches, with details that were obviously missing. Nanny wondered if he was producing only a partial view of a more complete picture that was somehow being replayed in his head. Sometimes the tune would disappear completely, leaving just the accompaniment. On other occasions he would play the melody alone, unsupported by any other parts. Nanny watched him closely and sometimes (only sometimes) she would see him hesitate as he worked out how to get *some* part of his hand (usually, though not always, a finger) on to the right note at the right time.

It amazed her that it wasn't just keyboard music that he could play. It didn't seem to matter to Derek whether the original piece had been performed by a band, a choir or even a full orchestra – he could still produce a creditable version of it on the Yamaha. In retrospect, we can surmise that it must often have been impossible for him to play exactly what he had heard, given the size of his hands, which could only just reach across five notes on the keyboard. So for him, whatever his inclinations may have been, performing wasn't just a question of playing by ear. It also meant he had to rearrange the music as he went along, in real time, so it conformed to his physical limitations.

It seems reasonable to suppose that this *necessity* to change things was an important factor in the development of Derek's musical creativity. From his earliest days at the keyboard, he was never just a tape recorder – or a 'human iPod' as he is sometimes known today in the States. As a toddler, where necessary, he would split up chords into their component notes so that he could manage to play these one or two at a time. He would reorganise music by putting the tune in the middle of the texture, divided between his thumbs, while his elastic fingers would add parts above and below – rather like a sandwich in sound. If, at any point, he judged there to be insufficient going on in a piece, he would liven things up by repeatedly striking a key or by filling in the intervals between notes with little scales: Derek's 'twiddly bits', Lord Patrick called them.

Gradually, as he became more fluent at performing a particular work, the texture would get fuller and more complex. Recordings of those early days reveal Derek able to create elaborate cat's-cradles in sound, with distinct melodic lines criss-crossing under and over each other – just like a kitten on the keys, thought Nanny humorously (now, whatever had made her think of that?) – miniature forerunners of the astonishing musical tapestries that Derek can weave today as a mature musician.

As a young child, though, the non-musical aspects of Derek's life were by no means straightforward. By the age of three, he was using a number of words, mainly to refer to people (his sister was known as 'My little Lib', for example) and everyday objects. However, he had the striking habit of 'echolalia': repeating whatever was said to him, rather than indulging in the usual give and take of childish conversation. He would repeat words and individual sounds obsessively – almost musically – as though the area of his brain that was trying to develop language had partly been usurped by the all-powerful desire to create patterns in sound. For him, words were playthings rather than the means to an end that most three-year-olds take them to be, and Derek couldn't use them effectively to make his wants and feelings known.

Understanding how one thing caused another to happen, and other concepts that children generally latch on to without conscious intervention on the part of adults, he just couldn't seem to grasp, despite Nanny's sustained efforts. Not being able to see obviously didn't help matters, but it was becoming clear to everyone that Derek must have learning difficulties of some kind. Perhaps the time in the incubator that had destroyed his eyes had affected his brain too? The family had never been warned of this possibility; though, if Derek were indeed intellectually impaired, it would explain some of the doctors' comments that they had only half understood before: the talk of 'developmental delay', for instance, and his probable need for 'speech and language therapy'.

Most astonishing of all, given his precocity on the keyboard, was Derek's inability to manipulate even the simplest of day-to-day items. No matter how many times Nanny showed him how to put them on and take them off, clothes remained a mystery to him. The use of any form of cutlery appeared to be a non-starter, and whenever she steeled herself to try again, the resulting mess was more than even Nanny could bear. As far as Derek was concerned, after two and a half years of handling them, toys were still objects to be struck together repetitively or to be fiddled with by his restless fingers. He seemed to have no idea that, in his imagination, they could turn into whatever he wanted them to be; 'pretend' play did not feature in his intellectual landscape.

Sensing that there was more to the world than he could understand, unable to express himself in words and having to rely on others to do almost everything for him was a recipe for frustration, and Derek would frequently explode with rage. With his face a deep red and the veins in his neck standing up, he would turn first upon himself, biting the back of his left hand until it was permanently scarred, and using his right to lash out at whoever was in reach. And if you tried to move out of the way, as those close to him soon discovered, he was surprisingly mobile and generally able to get where he wanted to be with uncanny speed. In fact, except when he was asleep or listening to something intently, Derek always seemed to be in motion: rocking on the spot, flapping his hands or weaving his head to and fro – a tireless bundle of nervous energy. Despite Nanny's long walks, which he loved, his only real release was through music. At the age of three, it was the cornerstone of his existence.

Christmas was approaching, Derek's fourth, and all were agreed that it was the logical thing to do. He'd managed brilliantly on the Yamaha, but now it was time for him to have a proper piano of his own.

Enthused by the idea, Nic phoned the proprietor of the local music shop. 'Something suitable for a child . . . Er, a three-year-old, actually . . . No, no, not a beginner.' He suddenly felt rather sheepish. 'Well, he can play classical, pop – just about anything really . . . Yes, that's right, three years old . . .'

The shopkeeper was used to dealing with parents who had delusions about their children, but Mr Paravicini was clearly in a league of his own. Still, a sale was a sale and, without probing too much further, the urbane vendor suggested that a Welmar upright would be just the thing: 'Robust? Yes, certainly!' (Whatever was this three-year-old like?) Why, he knew someone who'd learnt the Brahms 2nd Piano Concerto on a Welmar . . .

The trip from piano showroom to nursery took a while to organise, but finally, in mid December, the great day arrived. Nanny and Ester had prepared a space at one end of the nursery and two burly men heaved the new acquisition up the steps from the kitchen and into place. 'Someone'll be along in a

month or so to tune it, ma'am,' one of them said to
Mary Ann as she signed the receipt. 'Needs to settle
in, you know.' And with that they were gone.

Nanny flicked the pristine wooden case over with
a duster and carefully raised the lid. Eighty-eight
notes gleamed back at her. Well, Derek should have
fun with *that* lot. It must be twice the size of the
Yamaha, she thought. The piano had come with its
own stool and, as Mary Ann and Ester watched in
eager anticipation, Nanny lifted Derek up on to it
and guided his hands forward towards the keys. 'It's
your new piano, Bumps. I hope you like it.'

Although he didn't say anything, within moments
it was evident that Derek liked the piano *very much
indeed*. He discovered straight away that it had quite
a different feel from the organ keyboards that he had
played and, uncharacteristically for him, the first few
notes of the 'Raindrop' Prelude (which Nanny had
requested) sounded rather diffident as he got used
to the new touch that was required. His diffidence
didn't last long, though. He quickly worked out that,
unlike his grandfather's organ and the Yamaha, the
harder he hit the keys, the louder the sound that was
produced. With a certain inevitability, then, the
'Raindrop' Prelude became increasingly unsettled as
Derek's playing grew in intensity, rather like a developing storm that feeds on its own energy: the louder
the notes sounded the more excited he became, and
the higher his level of excitement the greater the
force with which he struck the keys.

To Derek, the effect was intoxicating and the
repeated notes of the prelude came to dominate

things to a far greater extent than Chopin had ever intended. More like hammer blows than raindrops, Nanny thought. Indeed, Derek's hands and arms even looked like hammers, she observed uneasily, as he somehow managed to clump all four fingers and a thumb on to each of the keys that he struck. His exhilaration was compounded by the discovery that the piano had far more notes than the Yamaha, and the raindrops gradually moved higher and higher up the keyboard, each note being given a thorough workout before he transferred his attentions to the next.

To the adults present the effect was distressing, physically painful even. Mary Ann uttered an oath and moved away from the piano; Ester put her hands over her ears; even Nanny flinched as the blows grew more powerful. It reminded her of the time when Derek had first tried playing the little old Parker-Bowles organ. Very soon, enough was enough. 'Derek!' she said sharply – though evidently, for once, without sufficient authority, since the raindrops continued to fall unabated. Derek had become obsessed with one of the white notes, about two-thirds of the way up the keyboard, which appeared to be suffering horribly, Nanny thought, as it was struck remorselessly again and again. (The piano tuner later informed her that it was the B two octaves above middle C.) 'Dere . . . ,' she started to shout, but before she could complete his name there was a sharp cracking sound followed by a dreadful twang, then a strange dull thudding as Derek continued to hammer away at the now useless note.

Mary Ann couldn't believe the truly awful scene that she'd just witnessed. Her little son, her vulnerable, blind, shouldn't-really-be-alive-today, three-and-a-half-year-old son, had single-handedly broken a brand new piano. 'Nanny!' she wailed desperately, in a voice that demanded 'Do something!'.

But Derek was already firmly in Nanny's grip en route to his bedroom.

When Nic learnt about the day's events later that evening, he simply couldn't believe it, and it was only after Nanny persuaded him to look inside the piano to see the damage for himself that he finally had to acknowledge what had happened.

He phoned the owner of the music shop the next day and *he* was incredulous too, though there was something in Nic's tone that warned him not to argue, and he promised to send a tuner out immediately with a spare hammer and strings, in case they were needed.

Lord Patrick heard about the incident the following Sunday and was *not* pleased with his godson, though it was impossible for anyone to stay cross with Derek for long. He took Nanny aside. 'What are you going to do?' he asked quietly.

'Well, it's the little organ all over again, isn't it? So the minute he starts banging, I'll just have to stop him playing for a few minutes until he learns. He'll get the hang of it all right.'

But Nanny quickly discovered that it wasn't as straightforward to keep Derek in check on the piano as it had been on the organ. With the old electric keyboards, whether he'd feathered the notes or thumped them, the same level of sound had still come out. So beyond getting Nanny's attention, there hadn't really been an incentive for him to hit the keys with more force. With the piano it was different, though, and Derek just couldn't help himself. After only a few minutes he became so engrossed with the music he was making that Nanny's admonishment to be gentle was invariably forgotten. Of course, while she was in the room with him a judicious clearing of the throat was enough to restore his playing to the mezzo forte range for a time, but she only had to go a little further afield, just down into the kitchen, for the volume level, and her hackles, to start to rise.

But Nanny persisted, as only she could, with infinite patience: day after day, week after week, month after month. In the end, an unspoken compromise was reached. Derek's playing, while loud (as it still tends to be today), remained within bounds *most* of the time and Nanny didn't feel obliged to rein him in so often. The frequency of the piano tuner's visits gradually diminished, Nic observed gratefully. When he did come, it was usually to repair the high B that Derek was so fond of (or did he dislike it? – there was no way of knowing), although after a couple of months he developed an additional penchant for F sharp below middle C, the tuner noticed.

Once the piano was mended, he would sit back with the cup of tea that Nanny always had ready for him and prepare to listen to Derek play. From where he was sitting, he could hear Nanny coaxing Derek up the steps to the nursery – 'One, two, three' – then guiding him along by the utility room. Finally he would burst in, rocking and fidgeting as ever, desperate to get going.

But Nanny would have none of it. *Manners maketh man*, and manners certainly came before playing the piano, as far as she was concerned.

'Good morning, Mr Sutton,' she would say, for Derek to copy.

'Good morning, Mr Sutton,' Derek would echo obediently, complete with Nanny's perfect diction.

Formalities over, Nanny would whisk him up on to the piano stool, tell him to sit up straight, neaten his hair with her fingers and urge him to play nicely (which Derek knew was code for 'don't dare bash the piano while Mr Sutton is here'). Then she would sit down herself with a well-earned cup of tea and look forward to being entertained.

'I think we'll start with . . .' she hesitated; perhaps best not to tempt fate with the 'Raindrop' Prelude so soon after the piano had been repaired. 'We'll start with "The Swan",' she said decisively. That was a reasonably safe bet. Nice and gentle. Usually.

As always, Derek didn't hesitate. Somehow his fingers went straight to the right keys and, in that instant, he was transformed. Where before had perched a severely disabled, unworldly child, almost totally dependent on others, there was now seated an independent, free-spirited young boy, confident in his own abilities. The seven octaves of the piano were *his* world, and he could explore and manipulate them as he wished. Here, *he* was in control.

To begin with, as though defining the limits of his territory and somehow instinctively knowing how to set the scene appropriately, Derek played cascades of notes right from the top to the bottom of the keyboard, then back up again. The effect of flourishes like these had been much improved since Libbet had shown him how to use the sustaining pedal, not really expecting him to understand. But to her surprise Derek had caught on immediately and, by sitting on the edge of the piano stool, had found that he could just reach to push the pedal down with the tips of his toes. This had opened important new possibilities for him, since it meant that for the first time he could keep the bass notes sounding while he played others above them – useful for all pianists, but particularly helpful for someone with such small hands.

Now, Derek's toe released the pedal as the mellifluous introduction came to an end and he introduced the swan, floating serenely on its lake of gently rippling arpeggios in the left hand. Andrew Sutton was duly impressed; Nanny was proud; and Mary Ann, who had just put her head round the nursery door, dutifully joined in the clapping at the end.

But Nanny could see from her face that she was worried about something, so, expressing a suddenly remembered concern that Mr Sutton might be late for his next appointment, thanking him for his efforts and voicing the hope that they wouldn't be seeing him again *too* soon (by now a standing joke between them), she showed him to the door.

Nanny hurried back into the kitchen. Mary Ann was somewhat distractedly holding an official-looking letter in one hand while flicking through the calendar on the wall with the other.

'What is it, Mary Ann?'

'It's the education people. They want a meeting to discuss Bumpy's school placement.'

Mary Ann had been dreading this. She knew from a previous phone conversation that a letter was on its way, but that was some weeks ago and she had hoped that somehow it had been overlooked. As she was to experience routinely over the next few years, however, the wheels of local authority bureaucracy grind slowly but inexorably – particularly where children are concerned.

She was worried about what they were going to suggest for him, but there was no choice. The traditional educational route for the family via public schools seemed out of the question. She couldn't imagine Derek on the playing fields of Eton (though he was subsequently to triumph there as a young pianist), and in those days schools were under no obligation to make provision for children who were blind or partially sighted, let alone those who had other disabilities. Hence the family were thrown back on to what the state had to offer.

Before the meeting, Derek apparently had to have an assessment from an educational psychologist, who in the next few days would ring to arrange a 'home visit' as the jargon in the letter had it. She would want to speak to Derek and have him undertake some simple tests. Mary Ann just couldn't imagine how Derek would respond and tried to blot the whole thing from her mind.

But all too soon the day arrived. Nanny welcomed the psychologist into the drawing room and offered her a seat next to Derek. She was neatly attired and carried a large black leather briefcase. He too was immaculately groomed and was sitting on the sofa in readiness for her visit. Sensing the anxiety in the air, he had started to fidget and now, uncomfortable with the stranger's proximity, his fingers were twisting awkwardly under and over each other. Nanny introduced Mary Ann, who was seated by the fireplace, and pleasantries were exchanged.

Then the psychologist turned to Derek. 'And what's *your* name?' she asked agreeably, thinking what a charming little boy he looked. She knew from her notes that Derek had been born very prematurely, but little else. Still, this should be a straightforward enough morning's work; she prided herself on having a natural rapport with young children.

'Derek,' Nanny replied forthrightly, partly to answer her question and partly so Derek knew to behave. She could sense the tension building up in him.

The psychologist looked across to Mary Ann, with a 'we're not going to get very far with *her* in the room, are we?' sort of look and Nanny was duly dispatched to make some coffee.

Once she was out of earshot, the psychologist leant forward to speak to Mary Ann. 'Who's she, exactly?' she asked confidentially, curiously.

'Nanny?' Derek called out, suddenly aware that she had gone.

'That's right,' affirmed Mary Ann.

Momentarily confused, but expecting more, the psychologist waited, pen poised over the form on her clipboard. 'Does Nanny have, er . . . a particular name?'

'Yes. Nanny,' reiterated Mary Ann in a vexed tone, uncomfortable with what she felt to be an unnecessary intrusion into their personal lives.

Embarrassed, the psychologist looked back at her form. There were three boxes, labelled 'title', 'first name' and 'family name'. Where should 'Nanny' go? she wondered. In the end she made a note in the margin to check out any details of Derek's relatives that might be held back at the office.

While they waited for the coffee to arrive, she tried to engage Derek in conversation, chatting about how nice it must be to live on a farm, with so many *real* animals. Did Derek know the names of any of them?

'Sefton,' said Nanny, re-entering the room with a tray of coffee.

She'd been quick, the psychologist thought, and hadn't really taken the hint. Or maybe she had. Then it struck her just what Nanny had said. Surely she couldn't mean . . .

Nanny put the tray down and picked up a framed photograph from the mantelpiece. Yes, it was true. There was Derek sitting on a blanket astride Sefton, with a joyous grin on his face, his whole body looking not much bigger than the horse's head.

The psychologist peered at the picture, confused. 'But . . . wasn't that the cavalry horse that was blown up by the IRA?'

Sefton had recently become a national hero for the stoical way in which he had coped with terrible injuries from the Hyde Park nail bomb. Since Andrew Parker-Bowles, Derek's uncle, was regimental commander of the Household Cavalry, it had seemed only natural that the horse should come to North Lodge Farm to recuperate.

The psychologist struggled to maintain her composure. She decided on a change of tack: some practical activities that Derek would be able to do easily and with which Nanny (hopefully) wouldn't be able to interfere. From a cloth bag in her case, she produced two plastic balls the size of small apples, one red and one blue, but in other respects identical. 'Here you are, Derek,' she said, placing one in each of his hands. They were hard and shiny, and he gleefully started to clatter them together. Nanny cleared her throat meaningfully. The clattering stopped and the psychologist continued. 'Now, Derek, are they the *same* or *different*?' she asked in an exaggerated way that made Nanny bristle. But the psychologist was focusing on Derek, confident that he would get it right. Since the balls felt exactly the same, the task was elementary.

There was an expectant pause while Derek very gently touched the balls together without actually clattering them. '*Same* or *different*,' he said, sounding uncannily like the psychologist.

The imitation – on this occasion not the sincerest form of flattery – was quite lost on her. 'Yes, I want you to tell me whether they are the *same* or *different*,' she intoned even more deliberately than before.

The woman's mad, thought Nanny. Doesn't she know he can't see? 'Different,' she said, unable to contain herself any longer. 'One's red and one's blue, Bumps.'

The psychologist glared furiously at Mary Ann, who all of a sudden seemed to have developed a singular fascination for the fire irons. Nanny just *sat* – unmoved, immovable.

There was a sticky silence, broken only by the steady squeak, squeak from the springs of the sofa as Derek rocked to and fro.

It was stalemate, but the psychologist had no choice but to go on. She had to come up with a report on Derek by the end of the week. She delved into her black bag again and this time produced a small shaker and a larger shaker, both of which she handed to Derek as a single item. Having no idea what she was giving him, he used both hands at once to get an awkward purchase on the two together. They weren't about to slip through his strong fingers, though, and the noise that they had started to make was pleasing, so he shook them both vigorously. Then wildly. Nanny cleared her throat again and the shaking subsided a little.

'Now, can you give me the *big* one?' came the wheedling voice once more.

Silently, Mary Ann implored him to get it right this time. But Derek held on to both the shakers tightly. Nanny cleared her throat so forcefully that it turned into a cough. Derek threw the shakers on the floor.

'Derek!'

Mary Ann could hear the final warning bell in Nanny's voice.

Hastily, the psychologist proceeded. 'Let's try something else,' she said. 'Now, do you know your mummy's name?'

By this time she wasn't really expecting a sensible reply from Derek, or from Nanny come to that. (The thought did cross her mind that perhaps she should be filling in a separate form for Nanny, but she quickly suppressed it.) Her pen hovered over the 'no response' box.

'Mary Ann,' said Derek promptly, distinctly.

The psychologist tried not to let the surprise show on her face. Instinctively, she probed again: 'And who's sitting next to you?'

'Nanny,' said Derek.

This time she did look surprised, gratified that at last there was something that she could tick off on her checklist. Nanny tut-tutted audibly. She didn't need a psychology degree to know that Derek had an excellent knowledge of his family and friends. Next to music, people were definitely his strength. He was not so good with *things*, though, she had to admit.

Her train of thought was interrupted by another question from the psychologist. 'And what do you like to do *best of all*?' she asked Derek, pen at the ready.

But Derek was distinctly agitated now and, tired of being made to conform, his left hand went up to his mouth and the other began to reach for the psychologist's hair.

Nanny, meanwhile, had read the signs just in time and, avoiding his outstretched fingers, had taken a firm hold of his right wrist. 'Best of all you'd like to play the piano for the lady, wouldn't you, Bumps?'

For the psychologist, what had until then been a very strange situation was now on the brink of becoming truly bizarre. 'You've got a toy piano, Derek?' she asked, struggling to understand what Nanny meant.

'No, a real one,' retorted Nanny brusquely and, without further ado, she led them both into the nursery.

Mary Ann breathed a sigh of relief as the tinkling of Derek's piano began to drift across the hall and into the drawing room. She dared to light a cigarette. Thank goodness for Nanny, she thought. She simply couldn't imagine Derek at school, having to manage without her.

An hour later, somewhat shell-shocked from having heard Derek's full repertoire fortissimo at close quarters and still reeling from the whole North Lodge Farm experience, the psychologist got back into her car and drove away from the house up the long gravel drive. As she departed, the geese honked and hissed angrily at her. She glowered at them. Slowly she went over the cattle grid and out into the road. Which way? In her confusion she couldn't remember. She had *never* had a morning like that before. And whatever was she going to put in her report?

The meeting with the Local Education Authority was always going to be difficult. Nic and Mary Ann, the Educational Psychologist, a social worker whom Mary Ann had seen from time to time, an 'Education Officer' and a further person whose function they never did glean gathered around a table in a dreary back room in County Hall. For a while the meeting seemed to drift. They went over how Derek came to be blind and what he had been doing at home. His 'interest in playing the piano' from the psychologist's report was noted. For goodness' sake, get to the point, Mary Ann thought, and she could see that Nic was feeling the same.

The Education Officer, who was chairing the meeting, fumbled with another sheet of paper. 'So, bearing in mind all we've heard, we've been thinking about which school will be best for Derek,' he said, doing his utmost to sound businesslike. 'Do you know "Westmead"?'

Neither Nic nor Mary Ann had ever heard of it. Maybe it was a primary school with a strong tradition in music.

'It's a special school – for children with a *wide range of disabilities*.'

The Education Officer started to describe the school, but Mary Ann could no longer take anything in. Nic was struggling too. Their son, at a school for disabled children? But Derek wasn't *disabled*, he just couldn't see and found it hard to understand things. With Nanny there, he was fine.

The rest of the meeting passed by in a blur and ten minutes later they were back outside, dazed, blinking in the strong daylight. The Westmead school prospectus dangled limply from Mary Ann's hands. They had been advised to 'read it at their leisure'. Any questions, please ring. And *do* arrange to visit the school.

When, one afternoon, Mary Ann and Nanny did eventually get to look around Westmead, they were initially pleasantly surprised. The head teacher was warm and friendly, seeming to understand their unspoken concerns. With evident pride, she led them down a brightly lit corridor that was covered with large paintings of farm animals that the children had been working on as part of their 'whole school project' (they should see our menagerie, thought Nanny). The door at the end had a sign on it that said 'Reception', painted neatly in large letters of different colours.

The Head knocked and partly opened the door. 'Visitors!' she trilled. 'Can we come in?'

Nanny's first impression was of light and colour and a bustle of activity, though on closer inspection she could only count five children – being assisted by three adults, she noticed. Mary Ann looked around the room and bit her lip. At the far side, by the French windows that led on to an outdoor play area, a little girl in a wheelchair was fiddling with some plastic shapes on her tray, encouraged by a smiling young lady in a blue T-shirt and jeans. Next to them a round-faced, dark-haired boy in calipers was whacking away at some plasticene on his table with a large wooden spoon. Another woman was sitting rather awkwardly on a low seat by his side, making what looked like plasticene candles, to go on his cake, presumably. Two other boys were fighting over a yellow plastic digger in the toy corner and a third helper was intervening, somewhat ineffectually, Mary Ann thought, trying to calm them down. She was sure that a quick dose of Nanny would sort them out! What were *they* doing at Westmead, she wondered. Finally, in a quiet area of the room, partly hidden by a small forest of paper lianas that hung from the ceiling, a girl whose head seemed much too large for her body was lying on a beanbag, staring vacantly upwards, not reacting at all to the action going on around.

Embarrassed to find that she was gaping at her, Mary Ann turned to the Head. 'It's all very nice,' she said, lost for words. But she was thinking, how on earth would Derek fit in? He was so used to Nanny helping him, interpreting the world for him, being his interface with other people, making sure that he didn't fall flat on this face – metaphorically and literally.

Again, the Head seemed to sense her concerns. Derek was to have one-to-one support, at least to begin with, to help him find his way around, get to know where things were, help him interact with the other children, play with toys and so on.

Nanny made some suitably positive noises for the benefit of Mary Ann but, deep down, she loathed the prospect of letting him go – releasing him into the care of someone else. He'd been her whole life for the last four and a half years and she feared that it was going to be as hard for her to move on as it would be for Derek.

Of course, when the time came, it wasn't as bad as everyone had feared. Derek began by attending Westmead three mornings a week, so to start with his time away from the familiarity of North Lodge Farm was in any case minimal. The staff at the school were kind and patient, and soon got to know most of Derek's idiosyncrasies. He got to know them, too, and seemed happy enough to leave Nanny at the classroom door and take his helper's hand. Every day he brought a 'diary' home, in which the teacher had jotted down a few notes to say what he'd been doing, how he'd behaved and if anything had particularly interested or upset him. Mary Ann, in particular, liked trying to read between the lines.

Monday, 10 September: 'Today Derek enjoyed free play outside in the sandpit.'

Now, what did *that* mean? Presumably that the contents of the sandpit had been dispersed over most of the playground. She could imagine the staff who had to sweep up the results of Derek's 'free play' enjoying it rather less than he had.

Wednesday, 26 September: 'In cookery, Derek helped Ami make some biscuits.'

But wasn't Ami the girl on the beanbag? The mind

boggled. How could Derek possibly help her to do anything? Anyway, Nanny had dutifully nibbled at one of the shapeless lumps that had arrived home in a Tupperware container and declared it to be delicious. Derek himself wasn't so keen on his own cooking, Mary Ann noticed, but he had enjoyed helping Nanny feed the rest to the geese.

Tuesday, 9 October: 'Derek had an accident with the drum in music today.'

Presumably code for the small pile of mangled wood and plastic that Mary Ann had noticed in the waste bin by the door when she had come to pick Derek up. She was concerned that school didn't seem to be taking Derek's music at all seriously – there wasn't a piano in the classroom and, despite a letter from her to the head teacher, written at Nanny's prompting, suggesting that Derek might perhaps be allowed to play the one in the hall from time to time, no action appeared to have been taken. The school piano, it seemed, was the preserve of the visiting music teacher who came once a week and played while the children sat on the floor and banged hand-held percussion instruments. The main aim was to get them to play when she played and stop when she stopped. No wonder Derek had bashed the drum, Mary Ann thought.

By Christmas, Nic was concerned too. Derek generally appeared to be happy enough at Westmead, but was he actually being *taught* anything? Shouldn't he be starting to learn Braille, for example? Nic phoned the RNIB, the main charity for blind and partially sighted people in the UK, with which he and Mary Ann had recently had some involvement in helping to organise a major fund-raising event. He enquired as to schools in Berkshire that specialised in the education of visually impaired children. There weren't any. How about schools in the South-East, preferably west or south of London? This time he got a positive response. There were three possibilities: Dorton House School in Kent, Linden Lodge School in Wandsworth, or Sunshine House School in Middlesex. They all seemed a very long way from Warfield, he thought. It raised the possibility of Derek having to board during the week and none of the family was at all keen on that prospect while he was still so young. But neither did they want things to go on as they were, so there was no choice but to take the next step and arrange visits to at least one or two of the schools that they had been told about. Which should they see first? They consulted a map and decided to start with the nearest. Linden Lodge it was.

Nic rang the head teacher – a Mr Matthews – to fix a date for them to look around the school.

The next chapter in Derek's life was about to begin.

Chapter Three

Hand in Hand

It was Wednesday morning after break and, as usual, I was giving Kelly a piano lesson. She was one of about seventy children at Linden Lodge, ranging in age from four to nineteen. About two-thirds of them, Kelly included, lived too far away to travel daily and so boarded at the school during the week. Having to stay away from home could be very difficult for the children and their families – particularly for the younger ones, like Kelly, who was only six. Of course, the staff did all they could to make things as homely and informal as possible, and the environment was pleasant enough: like so many residential special schools, Linden Lodge had been developed around a stately home, in this case an imposing mock-Tudor pile designed by Lutyens in the 1930s. 'North House', as the mansion was known, was set in ample grounds amid the green and leafy suburbs of SW19, within earshot of the Wimbledon tennis courts. It had been adapted for use largely as bedrooms for the senior pupils, with some classrooms and administrative areas. A further group of school buildings, incorporating purpose-built teaching areas, dormitories for the younger children and residential accommodation for some of the staff, had been added nearby in the 1960s. Their four-square, functional appearance, including flat roofs, faded cladding and metal window frames, looked rather incongruous alongside the fine brick-work and famous sloping walls of their distinguished architectural cousin. Inside, though, the rooms were spacious and light, and made a pleasant environment in which to learn. Kelly and I were in a teaching area known as the 'small hall', which was largely given over to music and other performing-arts activities.

Kelly was fun to work with. She had a good ear and I was helping her to pick out some tunes that she knew, using her right hand. Once she had a melody under way it was my job to provide a suit-able accompaniment. We'd played through a couple of spirituals and were just about to embark on the second chorus of Abba's 'Super Trouper', when I heard the door behind us click and, like it or not, I knew that we were about to have an audience. Not that either Kelly or I minded: visitors were a fact of life for us, as they were for the staff and pupils in many special schools – teachers in training, nurses, therapists, psychologists, education officers, prospective parents – and we were proud of what we did. It was nice to be able to show off.

There was no standing on ceremony at Linden Lodge, so we carried on without paying too much attention to the visitors – though out of the corner of my eye I noticed Mr Matthews accompanied by a rather tall couple standing somewhat awkwardly, formally, in the entrance to the room ('new parents,' I thought). Kelly, aware of the added attention being paid to her efforts, had started singing – 'Super Trouper beams are gonna blind me.' I felt a tingle of embarrassment and concentrated intently on our playing, not wanting to make eye contact at that moment. But suddenly, without warning, there was a distinct squeal – almost a shriek – and I felt something (someone?) push me in the back.

I half turned. It was a boy, a small boy I hadn't noticed before, mop of blond hair rocking back and forth, a bundle of daemonic energy struggling to free himself once more from his father's grasp.

'Sorry,' a cultured voice spoke from some distance above us. 'I do beg your pardon.'

But Frank Matthews was smiling and he started to say something to the visitors. They were momentarily distracted and, sensing his opportunity, the boy pressed ahead once more, undeterred, this time catching Kelly squarely in the back. Her impromptu performance came to an abrupt halt.

'Derek!' It was his mother this time, mortified with embarrassment.

'Don't worry. Are you all right, Kelly? Move along. We've got a visitor. Up you come, Derek.' And, amused, I lifted him into the air – he barely seemed to weigh anything at all – and plonked the wriggling mass down on the piano stool between us.

Immediately, like someone possessed, he attacked the keyboard, a frenzy of fingers, knuckles, thumbs, karate chops ... even his elbows were pressed into service, I noticed. I tried not to laugh.

Again, his father was speaking: 'Sorry. He's already broken our piano at home . . .'

But I wasn't paying attention. For it dawned on me that, despite the chaotic cascades of notes, he might actually know what he was doing. And yes, there, unmistakably, hidden within a dazzling kaleidoscope of sounds, were the strains of 'Don't Cry for Me, Argentina'. Instinctively I tried to join in, adding a bass-line. A left elbow was redirected towards me. Taking the hint, I tried an octave lower. I was caught by a karate chop.

This time I did laugh out loud: I simply couldn't believe what I was seeing and hearing. Clearly Derek wasn't used to sharing *his* piano with anyone else. His single-minded determination to play was extraordinary and I could only guess at the hidden depths of his musical potential. Yet his technique was the most eccentric I'd ever encountered – he must surely have been self-taught, though maybe now he was having lessons.

'Does he have a teacher?'

Derek's father gave me a quizzical look. Evidently I hadn't learnt from the karate chop. 'No. Er . . . we don't think he's ready yet.'

I could see what he meant. Teaching someone who wouldn't allow anyone else to touch the piano posed a real challenge. On the other hand, unless someone straightened out his fingering, indeed, his fingers, very soon (and, given the strength of his personality that was likely to be a considerable task) there was a real danger that the development of his talents would be for ever trammelled by the foibles of his unorthodox technique. It didn't matter how 'musical' he was: most of the piano repertoire had not been designed to be playable with knuckles and fists. And while such idiosyncrasies were diverting at the age of five, they would be less so by the age of ten, and downright odd by the time he was sixteen and a young adult. Action was needed now.

'It's never too soon to start,' I heard myself saying, my mantra to all parents, though the words sounded a bit hollow. Where would you begin trying to teach Derek?

I could sense that Mr Matthews was keen to move on to the next leg of his guided tour, though I couldn't imagine Derek being too interested in the science lab, the art room and the rest.

'Derek can stay here if you like. Pick him up on your way back. If you don't mind, Kelly?' I said guiltily, remembering that it was supposed to be her lesson.

Kelly, easygoing as ever, didn't mind at all, and she and I were royally entertained for the next half-hour or so. Derek seemed to know every piece she could think of and, provided that neither of us tried to join in, he was happy.

Of course, he made a huge fuss when the party returned and it was time to go, so there wasn't the opportunity to talk further. No matter, I thought. Mr Matthews will have their details and I can catch up with them in due course. I wanted to speak to them because by then I'd made up my mind. I was going to offer to teach Derek myself.

It was a few days before I had the chance to ask Mr Matthews for their particulars. No problem, he said.

He'd written down their name and address on a piece of paper that should be in his in-tray. I tried not to let my anxiety show, but the Matthews in-tray was notorious for being an administrative black hole into which letters, memos, circulars – anything that didn't require his immediate attention – disappeared, never to see the light of day again. And my concerns were justified when, the following morning, he sheepishly confessed that the vital piece of paper was missing.

Keen to make amends, though, he racked his brain and at last managed to remember part of the family's surname: 'It was "Para" something or other.' He frowned and pursed his lips. 'Para . . . Paravicini. That was it.' He'd thought it sounded Italian, Matthews recalled, but Mr Paravicini had told him that it was actually a Swiss appellation.

'Anything else?' I asked hopefully. 'Any idea where they live?'

More brain-racking, but no luck this time.

I tried not to let my frustration show. He was, after all, my boss. 'Any clues at all?' Without some more information the chances of being able to track Derek down – even with his unusual surname – seemed remote.

Mr Matthews smiled wanly, but my disappointment must have shown and he screwed himself up to make one final effort. There was a moment's silence and then . . . 'Tanks,' he said suddenly. 'Tanks. That's it!' He looked very pleased with himself.

I could feel the usual protocols of the teacher–headmaster relationship becoming strained. 'Tanks?' I queried. 'You mean they live near tanks, or . . .'

'No, no,' Matthews interrupted, 'Mr Paravicini told me that his company has something to do with tanks.'

'Right. Water tanks, or . . .'

'It begins with "s". Tanks or armoured cars. That's definitely it. In London somewhere.' And with an air of self-congratulation he strode off.

It wasn't until the evening that I had time to attempt to solve the riddle. I wandered into the school library, which was largely devoted to Braille volumes, though there were a few books in large print for the children with enough sight to read them. I eventually found one entitled *Vehicles of War* and flicked through the pages, searching for inspiration. The book had illustrations of two armoured cars that began with 's', the 'Saladin' and the 'Saracen', and one of the 'Sherman' tank.

I cross-referenced this unlikely trio with entries in the London business directory, and spent break times over the following few days making a succession of surreal phone calls to East End security firms, a property company, a cycle shop and various other enterprises – none of whom had ever heard of a Mr Paravicini. In the end, I had to admit defeat. It seemed, despite my best efforts, that I wasn't destined to see Derek again.

A few weeks passed and, although I hadn't forgotten about Derek, he was no longer in the forefront of my mind. It was the weekend and I was alone in North House, toying with an old crossword. Just one clue left: 6 down – 'Sounds like downpour's holding sway'. Eight letters: 'r', blank, 'i', blank, 'n', blank, 'n', blank. Hmm. Not too difficult: the answer must be 'reigning' . . . sounds like 'raining'. I put down the paper and yawned, thinking about nothing in particular. But I was still in the mood for puzzles and my mind was drawn back to the Paravicini riddle, as I now thought of it. Fictional detectives came to mind. My favourite was Miss Marple. What would she have done? Go over exactly what it was that Mr Matthews had said, no doubt: 'Mr Paravicini told me that his company has something to do with tanks . . . It begins with "s" . . . Tanks or armoured cars.'

I half remembered a Miss Marple story in which a witness had heard the name of the drug 'pilocarpine' but, not really understanding what it meant, had recalled it as a 'heap of fish'. Now, Mr Paravicini had told Matthews the name of his company, and it began with 's' – but suppose it *sounded like* the name of a tank or an armoured car: somehow, I just couldn't imagine Mr Paravicini being involved in the sale of steel-plated military vehicles. What were the possibilities? I went down into the school office and retrieved the phone directory. 'Saracen' seemed to be the most promising for alternative spellings. How about 'Sarasan', 'Sarasen', or 'Sarasin'? I thumbed through the 'S's. No, no, *yes* – there it was, *Sarasin Investment Management*. Well, there'd be no one there now; it was a Saturday. My hunch would have to wait.

I fumbled with the scrap of paper on which I'd written down Mrs Paravicini's instructions telling me how to get to North Lodge Farm: 'Just go straight through the Park, turn right, then left, then bear right on to Forest Road and *keep going*. Winkfield Row. We're on the left. Second entrance.'

I had managed to ascertain from her that she meant 'Windsor Great Park', but apart from that I had no further details. Anticipating problems, I'd allowed a couple of hours to get there from Wimbledon, never really expecting it to take that long. Now, an hour and forty-five minutes into the trip, I'd managed to locate a village called Winkfield (to which I invariably seemed to return) having skirted round the Ascot racecourse a couple of times.

It was a Sunday early in February 1985. An ice-cold wind was blowing that didn't meet much resistance from the ill-fitting window seals of my old green Triumph Vitesse and the windscreen wipers were no match for the snow that was now swirling around the car. I shivered and pondered Mr Paravicini's polite reply to my offer of lessons for Derek . . . Thank you. But would I wait until after Christmas because the piano needed 'some adjustment'. I wondered what he'd meant. Did I recall him saying that Derek had *broken* his piano? Surely not; I must have misheard.

A road sign seemed to appear from nowhere through the snow saying 'Winkfield Row'. At last. Along Locks Ride, then left into Forest Road and there, two minutes later, was North Lodge Farm. Consulting my piece of paper once more, I turned into the second of the two entrances. The cattle grid gave the Vitesse's worn universal joints a merciless workout and their clonking continued up the long gravel drive. A number of large saloons were pulled up in front of the house and I wondered where it would be politic to park. There was a stable yard to one side but that didn't seem right, so in the end I edged the Vitesse in between a large Mercedes and a BMW.

I took a deep breath, readying myself to confront the chilly afternoon air and the prospect of entering the Paravicini home. I felt strangely awkward foisting myself on the family. Did they really want me there or were they just being polite? What were they expecting me to achieve with Derek? Not too much too soon, I hoped.

You had to slam the driver's door of the Vitesse to get it to close and, as I did so, a large flake of rust fell off the wing and on to the snow that was starting to settle. Then I remembered the oil leak. Within an hour or so an unsightly black puddle would have formed under the engine. That wouldn't look good on the neatly raked gravel. Oh well, I'd be gone before they noticed and in any case perhaps they wouldn't want me back again.

I walked up to the imposing entrance to the house with its Georgian-style columns, guarded by two imperious-looking stone dogs and a more down-to-earth bristly hedgehog boot cleaner.

The bell was answered by a lady who, I judged, must have been in her late sixties, although there was a vitality in her face that belied her years. She greeted me with a polite smile and spoke with effort-less assurance: 'Mr Ockelford? Good afternoon. Do come in. I'm Nanny. Bumpy's waiting for you.' From

behind a pair of thick-rimmed glasses two percep-
tive eyes met mine, leaving me in no doubt that their
owner didn't suffer fools gladly. I wondered what
her initial assessment of *me* was.

I was ushered through a hallway dominated by a
large wooden staircase that wound its way up
towards the top of the three-storey house. A series
of fine old paintings of horses adorned the walls. We
walked past the dining room on the left. The door
was ajar, allowing the babble of after-lunch conversation and laughter to spill out into the hall. Nanny
led the way into a traditional kitchen, warm and
homely from the heat of the Aga, with the smell of
cooking still lingering in the air. Derek was there,
smartly kitted out in white trousers and a blue
sweatshirt, standing in the middle of the room,
rocking and fiddling with his hands. I doubted that
he would remember me, though he did seem to be
excited about something.

'Bumps! Come and say "Good Afternoon" to Mr
Ockelford.'

'Please, call me "Adam",' I said, before Derek had
a chance to respond. Most children found
'Ockelford' too much of a mouthful.

'Good afternoon, Adam,' enunciated Nanny for
Derek to copy.

'Good afternoon, Adam,' repeated Derek,
sounding just like Nanny but an octave higher.

'Hello, Derek. Shall we play the piano?'

'Play the piano,' he punted back.

I took that as affirmation, though it wasn't entirely
clear. So far, I'd heard him say very little, and then

only to repeat what someone else had just said. I wondered where the piano was, but Nanny had already taken Derek by the hand and was leading him through the kitchen, up a couple of steps, past a utility room on the right and into what she referred to as 'the nursery'. I looked around me. There were more pictures of horses, I noticed, and some of pigs, too. The smallish room had a comfortable sofa, a television and a stereo system built into a cupboard, a polished wooden rhino for children to play on, a box of toys neatly stashed away in one corner and, along the near wall, the subject of our quest: a modern upright piano. It didn't look damaged to me – at least, not on the outside.

Nanny lifted Derek on to the piano stool. 'Now, I expect Adam would like to hear some Beethoven, wouldn't you, Adam? How about the "Cantabile"?' Nanny had the knack of making questions sound like instructions.

A dining-room chair had been placed expectantly a few feet away from the piano stool (a precautionary measure? I wondered) and Nanny ushered me over to it.

I was curious to know what she meant by the 'Cantabile', but very soon found out as Derek started to play the slow movement of the *Pathétique* sonata. He began in A flat major, as Beethoven had intended, reinforcing my view that Derek must have 'perfect pitch'. This meant that whenever he heard a piece of music, the notes didn't just sound vaguely 'high' or 'low', as they do to most of us. For him, each one had its own distinct character.

This gave Derek a huge advantage as he taught himself to play by ear, since he didn't have to fumble around on the keyboard, finding out what sounded right by trial and error. Before his fingers even touched the piano he already knew which notes he needed to play. All he had to do was to direct his fingers to the correct key at the appropriate moment and the process was complete. Of course, being blind, this in itself was no inconsiderable achievement. Nonetheless, without perfect pitch it is doubtful whether his piano playing would ever have got off the ground.

At first Derek adhered more or less to the composition that Beethoven had written down for posterity – albeit a rather lumpy rendition with his own unique combination of thumbs and knuckles. But by the time the tune came round for the second time, Derek was starting to break away from the constraints of the accompaniment that Beethoven had provided and was adding extra notes to the left hand in particular. More like Chopin, I thought. The volume started to rise as more and more notes came piling in. Repeated chords appeared in the right hand. Liszt had arrived.

'Tea?' enquired Nanny, raising her voice to be heard over what was now a far from 'cantabile' piano sound.

'Thanks,' I mouthed back.

She returned to the kitchen.

At last I was alone with Derek – though probably not for long – so I decided to take my chance while I could.

As I had done at Linden Lodge, I reached forward and this time as gently as I could, started to improvise a bass-line below what he was doing. The notes were barely audible to me, but Derek was on to them immediately. His left hand shot down to where my fingers had trespassed, shooed the intruders away with a flick and instantly picked up from where I had left off.

Round One to Derek.

Leaving my chair, I walked over to the other side of the piano and started improvising an ornamented version of the tune high up – as far away as I could from his right hand. In a flash he was there again, pushing my hand out of the way. Then once more he began imitating what I had just played before extending it to fit in with the changes in harmony.

End of Round Two and Derek was clearly ahead on points.

Still, by following me to the extremes of the keyboard, he had left the middle range of notes temporarily exposed and, surreptitiously leaning over Derek's shoulders, with a feeling of mischievous triumph, I started to add in some chords. My victory was short-lived, however. Without for one moment stopping what he was doing, he tried to push me away with the back of his head. This time, though, I was minded to resist.

'Do you mind if I join in, Derek?'

My words fell on deaf ears. Ignoring me, he pushed with increasing force, all the time continuing to play. His message was unequivocal, so I decided to let him have his own way. For now. As soon as the coast was clear, his hands darted back to the middle of the piano, to fill in the chords that were now missing, before scampering outwards again to catch up with the abandoned tune and bass-line.

'You need an extra hand, Derek,' I joked, as in my mind I conceded Round Three to him. By a knockout.

Then Nanny was back with a pot of tea, two cups and some biscuits on a tray. 'How's it going, Bumps?' she asked.

Derek smiled at the sound of her voice, and the 'Cantabile' ended climactically in a way that Beethoven would scarcely have recognised.

'That was lovely. Thank you, Bumpy.' She started pouring the tea. 'Now I expect Adam would like to hear "Clair de lune".'

Beethoven-à-la-Derek was replaced with Debussy in similar style. I sipped my tea and munched ruminatively on a biscuit, wondering what to do next. Teaching Derek was going to be hard enough. Taking on Derek *and* Nanny was going to be a far greater challenge.

Still, the allotted hour flew by. Nanny suggested pieces to Derek that she thought I might like to hear and Derek performed them in his own inimitable way. Occasionally I tried to supplement what he was doing with extra notes or chords, but he was always on to me in an instant, trumping whatever card I played from his own deck of musical imaginings.

Nanny just listened approvingly without trying to intervene.

Finally, she glanced at her watch. 'We'll have one more, Bumps, and then it will be time for Adam to go. What shall we have? I know. How about "A Nightingale Sang in Berkeley Square"?'

Well, that made a change: at last a piece without a classical pedigree! Nanny sang along – Derek didn't try to prevent *her* from joining in, I noticed – though I comforted myself with the thought that she wasn't encroaching on what he considered to be *his* domain, the piano. And he followed the vagaries of her singing very well, even changing key at one point to accommodate her inability to hit the higher notes.

With Nanny leading the way to the end, 'I know 'cause I was there, that night in Berkeley Square', Derek's playing for once concluded calmly and quietly, and I had to admit to being quite moved.

'There, that was a lovely lesson,' said Nanny warmly. 'Now, say "Thank you, Adam".'

'Thank you, Adam,' Derek duly echoed, though I wondered whether I'd made any impression on him at all.

Nanny saw me to the door. The lunch party appeared to have broken up, most of the cars had gone and all was quiet. 'Shall we see you at the same time next week?' enquired Nanny. For some reason – and I really couldn't think why – I seemed to have won her approval.

I nodded.

And that was that. I couldn't help smiling to myself as I got back into the car. What *had* I let myself in for? Derek was every bit as magical as I had remembered. But how I was ever going to teach him anything, especially with Nanny there, I simply had no idea.

I put the key in the ignition and prayed that *my* old lady wouldn't play up. The cold and the damp didn't suit the Vitesse at all and I felt sure that the Paravicinis wouldn't welcome the sound of an engine being turned over for several minutes right next to their drawing room. So I felt a huge sense of relief as the straight-six immediately fired into life. The light was fading and I switched on the headlamps as I headed down the drive. The snow had turned to rain and the wet gravel glistened in dual beams of light.

With any luck, the oil slick would be washed away by the morning.

Those who had got to know Nanny well over the years, notably the Parker-Bowles family and their friends, had come to realise that she had a number of constant companions – guiding lights in her life. Among these were her own 'three Rs'. First, *religion*. Nanny had an unquestioning faith, inextricably linked to a profound love of life and a framework of unswerving moral values that guided all her actions. *Respect* was second, which for Nanny found expression in old-fashioned good manners and adherence to the common courtesies, come what might. Third was *routine* – for Nanny, orderliness was close to godliness – and it was this principle with which I initially became acquainted.

When I arrived at North Lodge Farm, Nanny would invariably greet me at the door and the same pleasantries would be exchanged. Without exception, Derek would be waiting in the kitchen, smartly dressed, rocking to and fro, and fiddling with his fingers in anticipation. Unfailingly, Nanny would intone 'Good afternoon, Adam' and, like clockwork, Derek would chime the words back. By then his hand would be reaching out ready to take hers as she led the way to the nursery. Every week she would lift him on to the piano stool, set him playing and go to make me a cup of tea. At each session she would determine the order of play and, when our sixty minutes were up, declare the innings closed before prompting the ritual thanks from Derek to his visitor.

At first, I found this hard to take; it ran against much of the prevailing philosophy in special education of promoting the personal development of children with learning difficulties by supporting them to make choices. If the locus of control was always with the adult, how would the child ever progress towards individual autonomy? But as I came to know what made the relationship between Derek and Nanny tick, I could see that there was more to their quirky alliance than first met the eye. Maybe, after all, intuitively she had got things right.

For example, it became evident that their interactions were far more two-way than the casual observer might imagine. Just who was in the driving seat? For sure, Nanny always seemed to be telling Derek what to do, but a moment's reflection indicated that *he* was actually pulling the strings more than she was. Quite without having any notion of what he was doing, he managed to command Nanny's undivided attention for virtually all his waking moments. It was *his* needs and *his* wants that drove practically all that she did.

Beyond this, I could see that the moment-to-moment structure that Nanny provided for Derek was a necessary step on the way to helping him make his own decisions. This was because he still appeared to find the world a bewildering place, which passed him by as a series of largely unconnected sensations, people and events, without the glue of understanding to hold them together. It struck me that Nanny's presence acted as a substitute for that 'glue' – not by enabling Derek to understand how things were connected, since his mind wasn't on the whole ready for that yet. But Nanny offered him the security that absolute constancy and consistency afforded. As Nanny herself later said, you can't make a meaningful choice unless you understand what the options are and what the consequences of your decision are likely to be.

All that seemed fine for now. But would Nanny sense when it was time to stand back, I wondered. Or would routine, for the time being the servant of Derek's development, become self-serving, inhibiting, the unintended master? That was an issue for another day: one that Nanny and I were to debate at length over the years to come. For now, she was everything to Derek: the conduit through which his experience of life flowed and through which other people interacted with him.

Gradually, though, my visits to North Lodge Farm began to evolve beyond the initial parameters that Nanny had set. For a number of reasons I switched to seeing Derek early on Saturday mornings and, when his hour was up, Nanny and I got into the habit of sitting together in the kitchen and chatting over a cup of coffee while Derek had some milk and a biscuit. Conversation flowed easily – partly, no doubt, on account of Nanny's honed skills as hostess and raconteuse, but increasingly through our shared interest in Derek, which was the catalyst for the respect and, in time, the affection that grew between us.

Through Nanny's compelling accounts, I formed a vivid picture of Derek's short history, of the precarious start to his existence, of his irrepressible fighting spirit in those first few days, weeks and months, of his eventual arrival home and of the early indications of his precocious musical talent.

She told me of her own eventful life, of growing up between the wars, of her decision to devote herself to the care of children as a professional nanny, of her extensive travels with some of the families for whom she had worked – including the experience of being on board a ship that came under enemy fire in the 1940s – and of her long and rewarding relationship with three generations of the Parker-Bowles family. I was fascinated to hear her perceptions of how the social order in England had changed during her lifetime and observed that while she spoke warmly of the years gone by, sometimes with a hint of nostalgia, she was never one for rose-tinted sentimentality.

Nanny might be firmly rooted in the past, I thought, but she lives for the present.

'And what about you, Adam?' Nanny enquired. 'What brings you to our door?'

I explained that I had recently taken up a full-time appointment at Linden Lodge as the Head of Music, having started out as a volunteer in the evenings when I'd been a student at the Royal Academy of Music in London. Then, I'd been fortunate enough to find one of the few landladies in the capital who, it seemed, positively welcomed music students – Eleanor ('Dickie') Ennals, former wife of the Labour politician and campaigner for human rights, David Ennals. Their second son, Paul (later to become a director at RNIB and Chief Executive of the National Children's Bureau), had worked at Linden Lodge in the late 1970s. Mindful of how musical some of the children seemed to be, he had suggested that I might like to get involved.

I had hesitated at first, wary of the potential commitment at a time when I was content not to have a particular direction in life. In the end, though, the prospect was one that I hadn't been able to resist, and I could clearly remember first approaching the school one autumnal Tuesday evening with a mixture of trepidation and excitement. Were some of the pupils really as talented as Paul had suggested? Surely he must have been exaggerating.

He had first introduced me to a boy called Anthony, who'd just transferred to the secondary department at Linden Lodge from another special school – Rushton Hall – which catered for the needs of blind children with additional disabilities. At the age of twelve, Anthony could play any instrument that he could lay his hands on, it seemed. The drums appeared to be his speciality, though he had also learnt the recorder, saxophone, clarinet and piano. Anthony had brought with him an LP that the pupils at Rushton had made to celebrate their musical achievements. The highlight was Anthony performing 'Take 5', playing both the saxophone and the percussion parts. This had evidently involved him in 'multi-tracking': laying down one part, then recording a second by improvising along with the first as it was replayed through headphones, a procedure that had been repeated a number of times to build up a complex texture in sound. Despite the concentration and control that this process must have entailed, Anthony's performance had a raw vitality, partly engendered, no doubt, by his attempts to play material that was at the limits of what he could manage technically. But what impressed me most was the immediacy of his playing: the apparently unstoppable urge to communicate through sound – something that I was to encounter time and again in my work at Linden Lodge.

Nanny listened with interest. I could sense that she was mentally trying to fit Derek into the broader picture that I was starting to paint. He was the first blind child that she had ever encountered and it was hard for her to know in what ways he might be typical or exceptional (although she had made a number of reasonable assumptions). I told her that, in my experience, Anthony and Derek were far from alone in their passion for music. At Linden Lodge, for example, there were some fine drummers in addition to Anthony, a group of guitar enthusiasts, a whole posse of proficient keyboard players and a gaggle of good singers. They regularly gave concerts in a range of venues, including local schools, clubs and care homes for older people. These were usually organised by Kevin Deegan, a teacher at the school, whose father, John, a fine musician who was himself blind, had taught there before him. He had been one of a number of important figures in Linden Lodge's rich musical heritage that stretched back in living memory to the celebrated jazz pianist George Shearing who had been a pupil for four years in the 1920s. Kevin, Paul Ennals and I became good friends, above and beyond our contact at the school – though it was the children who really had us hooked.

They had such a natural, unpretentious approach to music-making that was a refreshing change to the strict modus operandi that I had learnt to adopt as a classically trained musician, where things were very definitely regarded as 'right' or 'wrong'. In those days the idea that professional musicians should actively seek to widen interest and partici-pation in the performing arts through education and community programmes was still quite new, and the environment at the conservatoires could be some-what stifling for those who didn't quite fit in the box. The values I encountered at Linden Lodge were very different. Here the most prized musical skills were the ability to learn pieces rapidly by ear and remember them indefinitely, it seemed, and the flexibility to perform under almost any conditions. For example, the pianos that we encountered on our travels were very often a semitone or more flat, requiring on-the-spot transposition skills. But above all, there was no doubt in my mind that the children tended to hear things in a *different* way and it wasn't only a matter of the sense of 'perfect pitch' that so many of them seemed to have (around forty per cent of those who had been blind from birth, I reckoned – a far higher proportion than at the Royal Academy).

'What do you mean, they hear things *differently*?' Nanny asked.

The story of Philip came to mind. He was a young boy who, like Derek, had been born prematurely, but who also had a severe mid-range hearing loss. Incredibly, though, he too had an uncannily accurate sense of pitch, proudly informing me one day, for example, that the piano in the small hall was a quarter of a semitone sharper than the one in his classroom. I decided to check it out, running between the two rooms while trying to keep the sound of the 'A' from the small hall piano in my head. I was astonished to find that there was indeed a slight difference in tuning, though whether or not it was exactly a quarter of a semitone I had no way of ratifying.

As well as possessing a fine musical ear, Philip – unlike Derek – had a love of numbers and the abstract patterns that could be created with them. Hence it came as little surprise to me (notwithstanding the fact that he was only seven) that he developed a keen interest in the works of J. S. Bach, the master musical logician. Bar by bar, I taught Philip several of the preludes and fugues from Bach's great set of forty-eight. These are challenging pieces for anyone to play and understand, but Philip was intrigued to work out how Bach would use one short theme over and over again, sometimes turning it upside down or even halving or doubling it in length, ingeniously intertwining the different versions together to make one concordant web of sound. No one made these arcane structures more transparent than the idiosyncratic Canadian pianist, Glenn Gould, and Philip was particularly taken with his quirky interpretations, listening to the LPs I had given him over and over again.

Philip was not without his eccentricities, too. One Friday, after several weeks of effort, he finished learning the ninth fugue from Book I of *The Well-Tempered Clavier*, as the first set of preludes and fugues is known. He agreed to practise it complete over the weekend at home and perform it for me the following Monday. When the time came, we were both delighted with the result. The piece was demanding to play, with some awkward stretches for his small hands, but Philip had worked hard and he cleared most of the technical hurdles without stumbling. The fugue drew to an end, concluding on a sustained chord that Bach clearly intended as a moment of stasis at the climax of the piece. However, for some reason Philip saw fit to add another note in the left hand near the bottom of the keyboard after the winning post had been passed.

'Very good, Philip,' I congratulated him. His playing had been as meticulous as ever. 'But' – I hesitated, sensing that I might be entering personal territory – 'what was that last E at the end for?'

Philip shifted uncomfortably on his seat without answering. I was perplexed. Evidently there was something going on here that I didn't understand. Philip must have known that the extra note wasn't in the original and he liked to get things exactly right.

Why had he done it, I gently asked him again.

Once more he was evasive, though he finally muttered something about '735' making him unhappy.

I felt that I was getting to understand less rather than more. 'What do you mean, Philip?' I persisted.

He finally spat it out. 'It's an *odd number* and I don't like pieces with odd numbers of notes – so I added an extra one to make it all right.'

Briefly I wondered whether this was some kind of elaborate joke. I looked at him, sitting there earnestly on the piano stool – fingers pressing hard on his eyelids, pushing right back into the sockets. (There was another similarity with Derek, Nanny!) Clearly he was being serious. I tried to think of an argument that would make sense to *him*. 'Presumably Bach *meant* the fugue to have an odd number of notes?' I asked, temporarily suspending my disbelief as to the composer's likely intentions.

But it was to no avail. Philip was insistent that odd numbers of notes made him uncomfortable and he just couldn't resist making them even.

Could he *pretend* to play another note, I wondered – just listen to it in his head?

No.

So in the end we compromised. From now on, when playing pieces with odd numbers of notes, Philip would add his extra one discreetly to a chord in the middle so that no one else would notice.

Nanny was fascinated by this account. Although there was no way that Derek would possibly be worried whether a number was odd or even (although he could chant '1, 2, 3 . . .' aloud all the way to 10, he couldn't reliably say whether he was holding one object or two), she recognised in him a similar tendency to be obsessive. And funnily enough, she recalled, Derek often *did* like to add an extra note with his left hand, low down, at the end of pieces. But for him, she had suspected that it was because he couldn't bear performances to be over, so he kept them going for just that little bit longer. (Later on, when Derek started playing with other people, I thought that he added notes to the end of things because he wanted to have the last word!)

I decided to tell Nanny a final anecdote about Philip to illustrate the full extent of his precocious yet eccentric musicality. Again, maybe this would help her to put Derek's talents in perspective.

By the age of eight, I told her, Philip had learnt a number of the preludes and fugues by Bach: a great achievement by any standards. But the 'forty-eight' were themselves becoming something of an obses-sion, so I decided to see whether I could entice him into pastures new: nothing too radical at first – in fact, given the whole landscape of keyboard music that was available, into a field that was stylistically only a short distance away.

'Hello, Philip. I've got a new piece for you today,' I said, with a slightly edgy cheeriness, as he came into the classroom. We were following our normal weekday pattern at Linden Lodge. It was 8.30 a.m. He'd just had breakfast and we had half an hour together before assembly.

He immediately looked uncomfortable.

'You never know, you might like it,' I joked, as I helped him locate the chair next to the piano stool.

I played the opening of a piano sonata by Mozart. The catalogue of his works referred to it simply as 'K 333' – a label that was wholly unsuggestive of the sonata's classical refinement and unpretentious beauty. Beneath the surface elegance of the passage-work, though, lay structural symmetries that were every bit as rigorous in their conception as any that Bach had devised, and I thought Philip would appreciate the subtleties of the sonata's construction: in K 333, as in most of his compositions, Mozart didn't wear his musical craftsmanship on his sleeve.

'What is it?' Philip asked suspiciously, when the piano fell silent.

I told him.

There was a pause.

'I'd really like to do another Prelude and Fugue.'

I wondered what tack to take. Attempting to lead Philip down a path that he didn't want to explore was, of course, possible and sometimes necessary. But I knew from experience that if he set his mind against it, the process of trying to teach him K 333 would be unproductive for both of us. Philip was quite capable of sitting in silent mutiny, lesson after lesson, if the mood took him, refusing to play anything at all.

I glanced at him with that sweet-and-sour mixture of fondness and frustration that Philip was uniquely able to arouse in me, and decided to cut my losses and go straight to plan 'B'. Saying nothing, I slid the book of Mozart sonatas to one side of the piano's music stand, revealing another, slimmer volume that was open beneath and started to play. It was the last movement of the *Italian Concerto* by Bach. I performed the first couple of pages and I could sense from Philip's stillness and concentration that he was absorbed in the music.

I stopped.

A pause, then a small voice said, 'How does it go after that?'

Without saying anything, I carried on to the end. I didn't like to point out that although the piece was by Bach (which I guessed Philip had surmised for himself), it was neither a prelude nor a fugue. At that point, though, Philip wasn't interested in finding out what it was called. He just couldn't wait to swap places with me on the piano stool and get going.

As was the case with all the pieces that he learnt, he knew, just by listening, which notes he had to play. My initial task was to help him with the fingering, one hand at a time, working in slow motion. Usually he would memorise a few bars in this way, which he was then able to practise on his own. The *Italian Concerto*, though, had fired Philip's imagination, and in his enthusiasm to learn the piece he had digested the first three lines by the time the bell went for assembly.

Evidently he must have spent a good deal of time that evening practising what he had memorised, working away on his own, no doubt, on the piano up in his dormitory, because the next day he was able to play the opening at a respectable tempo. And he was eager for more, soaking up the rest of the first page like a sponge.

Philip maintained his focus and determination for the next month, by which time the three minutes or so of music had been committed to memory. The piece was technically demanding, comprising a rapidly flowing stream of notes that moved between the hands, and he needed ongoing assistance with some of the trickier twists and turns. Generally speaking, though, the continuous motion suited Philip's nimble fingers well and he gave a sparkling first performance during one Friday's whole-school assembly.

Of course, to sound at its best, I mused, as I listened to him, the music really ought to be played on a harpsichord, as Bach had intended. A thought stirred in my mind and that weekend I contacted my old harpsichord teacher at the Royal Academy, Virginia Black.

She listened carefully to my account of Philip's playing.

Yes, of course she would love to meet him and he would be welcome to visit her at the Academy ...

Finally, the great day came. Philip had been a

bundle of excitement and anxiety since breakfast time, and he hadn't been able to stop fidgeting on the tube on the way to Baker Street. I had tried to keep his mind occupied. What had he been doing over the weekend?

He told me that he'd been experimenting with a new tape recorder that he'd recently acquired. This meant that he now had two machines and could 'overdub' himself by playing along with what was on one while recording the combined effect on the other. That way he could build up a whole orchestra of Philips, all playing the piano at once.

'Right,' I said, in a 'that's interesting' sort of voice. I could picture the scene exactly, though at that moment I was more concerned with making sure that we didn't miss our stop.

And the funny thing was, he went on, the new tape recorder played back exactly one semitone higher than it recorded . . . (There must be something wrong with one of the motors, I thought, without saying anything, as I stood up ready to change at Victoria, but Philip was still talking, oblivious to the practical needs of the moment.) . . . So anything that was in F sounded as though it was in F sharp, and then he could re-record *that* in G, and so on, and the pieces got faster and faster . . .

'*Philip!*' I interrupted, worried that he would miss his footing and fall down the gap between platform and train.

In retrospect, I wished I'd listened more carefully to what he was saying, and its potential import for what was to follow. Looking back, it should have clicked that the *Italian Concerto* was in F, and that *that* was the piece he had been subjecting to his pitch- and time-warping experiments.

But none of this penetrated my consciousness as Virginia and I, ourselves excited and not a little intrigued, watched to see what would happen as Philip reached out and felt the compact keys of the double-manual harpsichord beneath his fingers. They suited his small hands perfectly and within a few moments he was instinctively starting to use the light but precise, almost mechanical action needed to make the quills pluck the strings cleanly.

'Well, do you want to give it a go, Philip?' I asked, when I sensed he had scrutinised the instrument for long enough. I sat back, smiled at my former teacher, closed my eyes and looked forward to hearing the assertive opening chords that Philip always managed so well.

As soon as he started to play, though, I could sense that something wasn't quite right. Surely, he was playing the piece in the wrong key? I opened my eyes and sat forward to get a better view of what Philip was up to. Yes, he'd started on F sharp instead of F. I didn't know whether to be more amazed that Philip had managed to pull off this extraordinarily difficult feat or the fact that he'd thought of doing it at all. To any 'serious' classical musician it was a truly bizarre undertaking. I was quite sure that nothing like this had ever happened before in the hallowed halls of the Royal Academy of Music.

I had to stop him.

Avoiding Virginia's curious glance, I put my hand

on his shoulder. 'Philip, what on earth are you doing?' Although my mind was racing, I tried to adopt an everyday tone – rather like an instructor speaking to a learner driver who had unexpectedly decided to pull away in fourth gear rather than in first.

Philip lifted his hands from the keys. 'Do you want to hear it in G?' And before I could reply, he was off again in the new key, and now at a discernibly faster tempo, I noticed.

This time I intervened immediately: 'No, Philip, no. We don't want it in G . . .'

He interrupted me: 'G sharp, then?' His fingers were already on the keyboard . . .

I could see that Nanny was agog with this story. Although Derek couldn't as yet say very much – and nothing at all about what he thought or felt – she could well imagine that his musical brain might operate in a similarly quirky way to Philip's. She had noticed, for example, that on one occasion when a Richard Clayderman tape had become caught up in the machine, the piece he'd been playing had become slower and slower, and more and more distorted, before finally grinding to a halt. For some time afterwards, it had amused Derek to play this mangled version of the Chopin.

'Doubly mangled, then, Nanny,' I said.

She looked at me blankly.

'Once by Clayderman and once by . . .' My voice trailed off. I could see that this first attempt at humour with Nanny wasn't going anywhere.

Luckily, her train of thought was already setting off down another set of tracks. 'So Philip was born prematurely, just like Derek, then?' she asked.

'Yes.' (Philip's family were quite open about his medical condition.)

Statistically, this was hardly surprising, for although Nic and Mary Ann hadn't realised it at the time, Derek was one of hundreds of children across the UK who were caught up in what was later recognised to be a national 'epidemic' of *retinopathy of prematurity* that began in the late 1970s. This went hand in hand with the increased survival rates of premature babies weighing less than a kilogram at birth. Of the fifty or so blind children who attended Linden Lodge in the 1980s, a staggering forty per cent had RoP. Of this group, a further forty per cent had learning difficulties. Almost all had a marked interest in music and half, like Derek, had 'perfect pitch'.

I could tell that it was these exceptionally musical children who really interested Nanny.

'So will Bumpy be able to play Bach like Philip one day?' she asked, for once slightly tentative with her enquiry.

I was honest with her. 'Derek's got great musical potential, Nanny, probably the greatest I've ever seen in anyone,' I said, fiddling absently with my coffee cup in its saucer. Then I looked her straight in the eye. 'But unless he'll let me help him sort out his technique, his playing's always going to be limited.'

There was a moment's silence. Her gaze met mine. 'And how are you going to do that?'

'Well, first he's got to learn to relate to *me* as a person in my own right.' I hesitated, then came out with it. 'I'll have to work with him on my own. Then, hopefully, he'll come to trust me, so that at least for some of the time he'll want to do exactly what I tell him.'

The implication was clear: in order for me to see inside Derek's head and show him the way forward, I would have to form a relationship with him that was comparable in intimacy and depth to Nanny's. Would she be prepared to let that happen? Would she be prepared to let go?

I could see her thinking about what I had said, so I pressed home my case. I assured her that the last thing I wanted to do was to interfere with the way that he related to other people through music or to inhibit the spontaneity of his playing. But it was only by acquiring a sound technique that he would ultimately be free to play whatever and however he wanted.

No more was said about the matter and I wondered if I had gone too far. Nanny had Derek bid me a polite farewell as usual, but it was impossible to know what she was thinking. Oh well, I would find out next week whether or not she was prepared to take heed of what I had said.

The seven days passed by quickly enough and before I knew it I was back at North Lodge Farm for another musical (and extra-musical) encounter.

'Morning, Derek,' I said brightly, as Nanny brought him to welcome me at the door. I put my hand on his shoulder, partly to make physical contact and partly in an effort to stop him rocking.

And so the ritual trialogue of greetings got under way. Nanny prompted Derek to reply to me and then offered me her own salutation, to which I responded. Then we started again. By the time the dizzying round of 'good mornings', 'how are yous' and 'very well, thank yous' was complete I was ready for my cup of coffee.

But this week I was to be disappointed.

'Right, Bumpy, I want you to take Adam through to the nursery. I've got some sorting out to do upstairs,' she announced. 'Play nicely, and I'll see you in an hour.' And she gave him a big kiss.

I was taken aback. I felt the urge to say something to Nanny, to thank her for understanding, for seeing the bigger picture. But I sensed that wasn't the form. There was no need to say anything – it would have been inappropriate – and anyway, Nanny was already in the hall, scooping up some papers to take with her.

So I turned instead to her young charge, entrusted to me for sixty minutes.

'Right,' I thought. 'Now I've got you, Derek, what am I going to do with you?'

I decided to start with some five-finger exercises, the foundation of all keyboard technique: just up and down the keys, one note for each finger and the thumb. Would Derek find that sufficiently engaging? How would he react? But these questions were supplanted in my mind by a more immediate problem: how was I going to be able to get at the piano for long enough to play the notes that he was supposed to be copying?

Sitting next to him on the piano stool, I tried holding both his wrists with my left hand to give my right free rein on the keyboard. I reckoned that I only needed about ten seconds. But that was nine too many for Derek. He wriggled out of my grip in no time and struck the C that I had managed to play before being overwhelmed. I was afraid of hurting him if I held his wrists any tighter, so I had to try something else.

'Right, Derek,' I declared, 'we're going to play a game. You're going to sit over the other side of the room while I play something on the piano, then you can come over and see if you can copy it.'

I didn't really expect to him understand what I'd said, but in any case, without waiting to see his re-action, I picked him up and plopped him down on the floor at the far end of the nursery. I strode back to the piano and quickly played the five-finger exer-cise. I'd only just finished when Derek, who'd been amazingly quick out of the starting blocks and had fairly scuttled across the room, was pushing me out of the way. That done, he reached across the stool and played what I had – well, a version of it. He used both hands to play a series of chords, up and down. I had to laugh at his antics.

Then he stopped, waiting. This was a game whose rules he had somehow immediately grasped.

So I picked him up again, sat him as far away from the piano as I could, raced back and played the exer-cise once more – this time starting on the next note up, C sharp. Again, my thumb was barely off the last key when Derek was back with his response.

And so we continued up the chromatic scale, until we'd tackled all twelve different keys. That brought us back to C and it felt right to stop there. Derek seemed to sense that feeling of completion too and was content to return to his familiar routine of taking requests for pieces to play. He still wouldn't let me join in, I noticed, but I didn't mind: I was convinced that the five-finger-exercise game had provided the breakthrough that I had been looking for. Now I had something to build on.

Driving home later that morning, I smiled as I mulled over what had happened and couldn't help wondering what my own childhood piano teacher – a staid, scale-loving spinster with a Siamese cat – would have made of it. She certainly wouldn't have regarded our unconventional interaction as a 'lesson'. But then, Derek had no idea of what it was to be 'taught', let alone how a 'teacher–pupil' relationship would normally function. These things were currently outside his experience. But somehow he was going to have to learn what they meant.

Next week, as soon as I suggested that we should play our game, Derek's hands reached out for me to pick him up. He'd evidently remembered what we'd done before and the five-finger exercises were now the first element in *our* routine. For me, the important thing was not putting Derek over on the other side of the room and having him find his way back to the piano (though that in itself was valuable practice in independent movement), but the fact that he was learning to listen and copy systematically within a defined social context. It soon became apparent that it was the music that really lay at the heart of things for Derek too, and by the time the five-finger exercises had traversed the twelve different keys, all I was having to do was pick him up and put him on my knee, and he was content to let me play before taking his turn.

It was then a short step in the lesson that followed to leave Derek where he was on the piano stool, and to engage in the 'play-copy' dialogue with no physical intervention on my part at all. In due course, I started to imitate what *he* was doing too, enabling us to have a genuine musical 'conversation'. And it wasn't just a matter of a musical ball bouncing between us like echoes in an alleyway. Whatever you lobbed at Derek would invariably come hurtling back with interest and it was challenging to keep up with his musical repartee, which combined wit and ingenuity with an incredible speed of thought.

With no words to get in the way, a whole world of sophisticated social intercourse was now opened up to him. It was the second 'eureka' moment of his life: having first discovered that he was able to play what he could hear, now he came to realise that he could communicate *through* music. Indeed, for Derek, music came to function as a proxy language, and it was through music that his wider development was increasingly channelled.

Despite the great strides that we had made in the course of only a few weeks, there were still huge obstacles to be overcome if Derek was to fulfil his musical potential. I decided that the next major challenge to tackle had to be his technique. Although he could copy the notes I played just by listening, he couldn't, of course, see how I held my hands at the piano, which fingers I used, and the fact that my elbows didn't figure at all in what I did. To plug this gap in his experience, I tried putting his hands over mine, one at a time, so that he could feel the shape of my hand and, to an extent, what my fingers were doing. We tried it for a few weeks, but it didn't seem to make any difference: whenever it was his turn, Derek just carried on as before.

So I tried a different approach. I held his right hand on mine.

'Look, Derek, here's my thumb,' I said, giving it a wiggle as his fingers curled around it.

'Now, where's yours?' I guided him to feel his right hand with his left.

'That's it! Now, let's put your thumb on C, middle C.' He allowed me to help him find the correct note and to push it down with his thumb.

'There you are.' And I sang 'thumb'.

Next I uncurled his index finger and placed its tip on D. He pressed the note.

'Second finger,' I sang.

And so we continued with his third, fourth and little fingers, before coming back down to the thumb. He sang along enthusiastically and couldn't resist adding in an accompaniment below. When we swapped over to his left hand, he treated the five-finger exercise like a bass-line and added tunes in the right. No matter, I thought. The main thing was that, for the first time in his life, he'd manage to play using something approaching a conventional technique. On that simplest of foundations we would subsequently be able to build.

Little did I appreciate at the time just how long Derek's technique would take to reconstruct. For a total of eight years we worked together, weekly and then daily, spending hundreds of hours physically going over all the basic fingering patterns that make up a professional pianist's stock-in-trade. From five-finger exercises we moved on to full scales: major, minor and chromatic, as well as some of the more exotic varieties – the so-called 'modals', the whole-tones and the octatonics. Scales had the additional complexity of requiring Derek to tuck his thumb under his fingers while his hand was travelling in one direction, and to extend his fingers over his thumb while it was coming back in the other. I had to use both my hands to help him get this action right. We also tackled arpeggios: major, minor, and dominant and diminished sevenths, followed by some of the more unusual forms – French sevenths, augmented triads and chords of the added sixth. Long after my threshold of boredom was a distant memory, Derek would be keen for more. There was something about the orderliness, not only of the scales and arpeggios themselves but also the regular way in which they related to one another, that he clearly found deeply satisfying.

I invariably told Derek what the scale or arpeggio that we were about to play was called, and he picked up on the names of the notes very quickly – even those that confusingly had two labels, such as A flat (which is also known as G sharp). Within a few weeks he had also got to know the meaning of the terms 'major' and 'minor', which in the West are traditionally associated with 'happy' and 'sad' music respectively. And that, somewhat to my surprise, was as far as Derek's grasp of music theory ever got. Every other type of chord was referred to as 'diminished' or occasionally 'diminished and diminished'. Not that a knowledge of such terms was at all important for Derek's playing, though from time to time it has made communication with other musicians problematic. Usually, though, they soon realise that it is best to indicate what they mean by showing him, rather than relying on verbal labels, which can have unpredictable results.

As Derek worked on the technical exercises, I consciously used other language in didactic ways too. For example, singing the name of each finger as it was used soon became an established habit. I hoped that this would help Derek forge the cognitive connections that he needed to develop a conceptual awareness of what his hands were doing. This would have a number of potential benefits: not only would learning the piano become easier, but his life skills should take off too. For despite Derek's dexterity on the keyboard, handling buttons, laces and belts remained quite beyond him.

However, in spite of the tens – perhaps hundreds – of thousands of willing repetitions, Derek never did learn to tell which finger was which. And even today, if you ask him to hold up his thumb (rather than his fingers), he still can't do it reliably, and the capacity to distinguish one hand from the other continues to elude him. While this seems odd – incredible, even – given his dazzling virtuosity, with hindsight I've come to realise that being able to put a name to concepts such as 'left' and 'right' wasn't the most important thing. What really mattered was achieving that very first aim I had identified when I initially watched Derek play: that his technique should develop sufficiently so as not to trammel his vivid aural imagination. And that, over the years, is exactly what *did* happen. During all those hundreds of hours of practice he absorbed many of the standard fingering patterns, quite without being aware of it, and these slowly became assimilated into his own playing. Today his technique, as a mature adult performer, although still far from conventional, enables him to do whatever his musical imagination demands.

My first year working with Derek at North Lodge Farm passed by all too quickly; the Christmas and New Year celebrations came and went, and January 1986 made its appearance on new calendars everywhere. I was delighted with Derek's progress and Nanny clearly was pleased too. We were now a team. I taught Derek two or three new pieces a week, leaving tapes for him to listen to when I had gone, usually a mixture of my own and professional recordings. Nanny organised Derek's practice sessions assiduously, making careful notes of what I wanted him to learn in time for the next lesson and making sure that he did it.

The issue of Derek's longer-term future was troubling me, though. It was now over a year since he had visited Linden Lodge and I had heard nothing more. I asked Nanny whether she knew anything and, for once, I felt that her negative reply was rather evasive.

What was going on?

I could imagine some of the issues that were having to be resolved behind the scenes. First, the Local Education Authority would have to pay considerably more for an 'out-county' placement than they did for Derek to attend Westmead School, and they could well be resisting having to find the additional fees. Second, I could sense that Nanny did not want Derek to board, so there may well have been some ongoing inertia there. I could quite understand it: Derek was still only six and a half and, especially given the nature of his other disabilities, she regarded that as far too young for him to leave home and be deprived of the special care and attention that she was able to provide.

But there was a third, and much more worrying, issue that I only became aware of by chance some weeks later. At a meeting of fellow music teachers working with visually impaired children, I overheard a colleague from Dorton House School in Kent talking about a remarkable young boy who had just attended for assessment. Truly amazing, she said. He could play *anything* that was asked of him. Rather wild, though! She paused for effect, letting her small audience imagine what form the wildness might take. I had to admit to being curious too. Very curious. Apparently, he never stopped rocking and poking his eyes and (her voice dropped slightly at this point) he had even tried to *bite* her when she told him it was time to stop! This drew an audible gasp from her band of worthy colleagues. She'd never forget him, she went on. A fine head of blond hair ...

Suddenly, I felt physically sick. No, no ... they couldn't do this, not after all that Derek and I had achieved together and with so much more to come. For one awful moment I wished Derek *had* bitten the teacher. My thoughts jumped around, trying to rationalise what I'd just heard. So *that* was why Nanny had been evasive. The family, prompted by the council no doubt, were evidently looking at other options. That would make sense, since at the time the fees for Dorton House, which was run by a successful charity, were significantly less than those for Linden Lodge, which only had local authority backing. The bottom line was, if Dorton said that they were able to meet Derek's needs – and, as a special school for blind and partially sighted children they surely would – then there was no question: he would be placed there. There seemed to be little doubt that my work with Derek was about to come to an end.

Chapter Four

Linden Lodge

I drove home from the meeting in a daze. I suppose until then I just hadn't realised how much of an emotional investment I had made in Derek over the preceding twelve months. I tried to add up what that commitment had become in day-to-day terms. I must have expended many kilojoules of mental energy as well as countless hours of time that went far beyond the Saturday mornings that had been taken up at North Lodge Farm – searching out particular recordings that I thought Derek would enjoy and that would extend his musical horizons, making practice tapes for him to work on with Nanny during the week, and simply contemplating what to do next. For at the end of every session with Derek I sensed that there was still more to come – a great deal more – and that I hadn't as yet come near to fathoming the depths of his labyrinthine musical mind. I was continually working out how to help him realise the next level of his potential. It was rather like trying to look round the bends in a tunnel that was twisting further and further into the ground, with a light flickering somewhere at the end. Every time you thought that you'd got there, it turned out that there was another bend to negotiate. Yet on each occasion, the light that appeared to be just beyond reach was brighter than it had been before: he was yet to show us the full brilliance of his latent musicality.

It was the ongoing challenge of this music–psychological exploration, with all its uncertainties, difficulties and unexpected delights, that for me was the real buzz of working with Derek. He was unique. To be able to work with him was a huge privilege and, without doubt, the opportunity of a lifetime for someone interested in exceptional musical development. It dawned on me that helping Derek to unlock his own kooky genius – to become fulfilled musically and personally – had become my vocation.

But realising this only made the prospect of handing over responsibility for Derek's music education to another person at this early stage all the more painful: it was too soon for him to move on. What, then, was I to do? I consulted my two closest friends and colleagues at Linden Lodge, Paul Ennals and Kevin Deegan. We chatted over a pint in our favourite pub, the Red Rover in Barnes.

We agreed that I had an overriding responsibility to act in Derek's best interests. But what did that mean in the current circumstances? I honestly felt that he would be better off remaining under my tutelage and coming to Linden Lodge. Nonetheless, Dorton House had many strengths to offer. In any case, maybe the two options weren't mutually exclusive. I could, perhaps, continue to play a part in Derek's musical education even if he were at a different school (which was, after all, what was happening at the time).

I decided to write to Nic and Mary Ann. I offered to go on supporting Derek whatever their decision, while expressing the view that it would be quite wrong for his future placement to be determined by the council purely on financial grounds. I felt that that was as much as I could appropriately do.

The weeks passed and there was no reply to my letter. I would have liked to broach the subject with Nanny, whom I still saw every Saturday with Derek, but the moment never seemed right. I had set out my position and now it was down to the family to decide what should happen next. It felt wrong to try to exert undue influence on what was, after all, a personal matter for them to negotiate with their Local Education Authority.

So my sessions with Derek continued irrespective of any thinking that might or might not have been crystallising behind the scenes. Spring turned to summer, and in July I had my first experience of a birthday party, North Lodge Farm-style, when Derek was seven. As ever, Nanny had everything and everyone perfectly organised and the afternoon ran like clockwork. Derek's family and friends turned out in force. His favourite part was accompanying his guests as they sang 'Happy Birthday', which he was keen to draw out for as long as possible. After four verses Nanny decided that it was time to get someone to assist Derek in what was for him the far more difficult task of blowing out the candles on the cake. Following that there was swimming for the hardy (the pool hadn't been heated for some time) and a game of 'big ball' for those who fancied more genteel exercise.

I was among a third group, for whom any exercise was anathema. We attempted to conceal ourselves under the sunshades on the veranda, sipping cocktails, but Nanny wouldn't have any of it. Only those who were too infirm or too inebriated to stand were excused. The rest were dragooned into a circle on the lawn at the back of the house. Nanny placed Derek in the middle with a large beach ball. Tisha Monson, one of Derek's godparents, initiated proceedings by calling to him to push the ball in her direction. With a deft flick of both hands he sent the light plastic sphere skimming over the grass towards her. She immediately batted it back into his outstretched arms. As soon as it made contact with him he grabbed hold of the ball again, slapping its springy surface with excitement while waiting for the next voice in the ring to call out to him. From his left, Libbet obliged, and again his aim was true. I was impressed. What a perfect game it was for Derek, enabling him to engage with other people – and, for once, in a non-musical setting.

His zest for the game and the summer heat soon wore down all but a hard core of players and, with the punchbowl beckoning, it wasn't too long before Nanny and I were the only participants left – standing in our customary triangle with Derek. My concentration drifted. If Derek were going to move school, then the forthcoming summer holidays would be the obvious time for this to happen. So, when term started in September, Derek wouldn't return to Westmead but would make the trip to Dorton House.

My reflections were broken by Nanny's sudden warning that the ball was drifting towards the hedge.

'Wake up, Adam!' she called out, in a way that made Derek laugh. Then, sensing that the game had reached its natural conclusion and that Derek needed to unwind, she added, 'Come on, let's go for a walk.'

Slowly, the three of us made our way down the drive and then, as our shadows started to lengthen before us, round the lake. By the time we had returned to the house, the last of the guests had gone and Ester had begun the long process of clearing up. We stood by my car.

'Have a lovely summer, Derek,' I said, trying hard to inject brightness into my voice.

Then I turned to Nanny. 'I'll give you a ring some time to fix a date for September?'

'That would be lovely, Adam.' Her perfect manners weren't just a veneer, they were Nanny through and through, and on occasions like this she was wholly inscrutable. I just couldn't tell whether she was aware of other plans being hatched for Derek or not.

'Goodbye, Adam, and thank you for coming to my party,' she intoned.

Derek duly echoed her.

I wondered what he was really thinking. At least he was unaware of the uncertainty encircling him.

'Goodbye, Derek!'

I gave the old car door the necessary slam, start-led the engine into life and drove off into the dusk.

The day before the start of the new academic year always sped by in a flurry of belated activity. I was in the music room at Linden Lodge, surrounded by piles of open songbooks, searching for inspiration on the theme of 'animals' for the whole school. The little ones would like 'Puff the Magic Dragon', no doubt, while the juniors would be amused by the 'Spanish Flea'. The older ones might enjoy grappling with 'Fish Gotta Swim, Birds Gotta Fly' and, yes, how about 'Karma Chameleon'?

There was a knock on the door and there was Maggy Grubb, just starting her second year as head teacher following the retirement of Frank Matthews. She held a half-folded bundle of papers in her hand. 'You'll never guess what?'

I couldn't guess. Perhaps the music inspector was coming in next week? I wondered again about the suitability of 'Karma Chameleon'.

Maggy smiled. 'No, no, it's nothing like that. Berkshire have asked us whether we'd be prepared to take Derek Paravicini!'

I was amazed, disbelieving and pleased all at once. And then overwhelmed with sheer delight. 'But how come? I'd heard he was going to Dorton.'

'Apparently not. They don't feel they can offer him a place. Hold on, I'll show you their assessment. It's attached to the back of the letter.' She leafed through the papers. 'Mmm. According to them he's got challenging behaviour – won't do as he's told, disruptive and a tendency to *bite*, apparently.' She looked at me questioningly. This account bore little correspondence to the picture I had painted of Derek over the previous eighteen months.

I felt a twinge of anxiety. 'They just don't know how to handle him. Provided he's with people he knows and things are structured so that he understands what's going on, he's fine.'

Maggy sighed. She could sense conflict looming. Derek's case was symptomatic of the transformation that was sweeping through special educational provision in the UK at the time and, as with all change, the metamorphosis was welcomed by some and resisted by others. Traditionally, Linden Lodge had catered for the needs of children who were unable to learn through visual means, whose preferred medium was Braille. However, by the mid 1980s, following the Warnock Report of 1978 and subsequent legislation, the position was becoming much more complicated. Increasingly, pupils who were 'only' blind or partially sighted were being included in the mainstream, and the function of special schools such as Linden Lodge was evolving to meet the needs of children, like Derek, who had disabilities in addition to a visual impairment. This was necessary since recent medical advances meant that an ever greater number of babies were surviving serious illness or trauma, which before would have proved fatal. But doctors' success was presenting society with a daunting legacy: tens of thousands of children with severe or profound disabilities who required a whole new range of educational, social and healthcare services. Hence our role in schools such as Linden Lodge was having to develop to keep up with the rapidly changing needs of our pupils. Whereas before advanced Braille skills had been the order of the day, now teachers were also having to learn how to foster verbal communication in children who were still learning to speak during their school years. PE and sport were gradually being supplemented with 'movement skills' and physiotherapy. And the notion of discipline was being replaced with behaviour management.

The problem was that the pace of change was outstripping schools' ability to deliver the new curricula. There wasn't a ready-made bank of resources and expertise to which one could turn when confronted with someone with very special learning needs such as Derek. They simply hadn't yet been invented or acquired. In my view, as far as these children (young people who would today no doubt be described as being on the 'autistic spectrum') were concerned, there was an awkward mutuality in our ignorance about them and their misunderstanding of us. It was little wonder that they should choose to bite us from time to time, I mused, since we were certainly cutting our teeth on them as teachers in this brave new world of education. To me it was obvious that we should be embracing children with complex needs and learning from them: they were our future.

This was not a philosophy with which all my colleagues were comfortable, however. And there had been one or two new entrants to Linden Lodge in the preceding year who had engendered a lively debate as to the school's admissions policy, which appeared to be changing by default rather than design. There was a strong view that we should wait for a while before taking on any more children with severe learning difficulties and behavioural problems in addition to a visual impairment. The nature of the school was altering too quickly, it was argued, and we didn't have the capacity to cope.

Inevitably, Derek appeared as an item on the agenda at the next staff meeting.

I listened as the view was expressed (from people who had never met him, I noted, with some annoyance) that Derek would be better off in an institution that specialised in educating children with learning difficulties and the management of challenging behaviour.

But how would they deal with the fact that he couldn't see, I wanted to know.

Was I really saying, then, that Derek's blindness was his main problem? If not, then Linden Lodge surely wasn't the right place?

It's not like that, I countered. The fact that he couldn't see and found it difficult to understand things interacted in a complex way. He needed *combined* expertise in order to thrive.

Was I saying that we had this expertise?

Nowhere yet had fully developed that expertise, I retorted. We should be seeking to lead the way.

And what about his tendency to hit out at people and bite when he was stressed?

I argued that we should work towards providing an environment that minimised his stress.

I could sense, though, that I was making little headway, so I went on to the offensive.

What about his music? Who was going to teach him if he didn't come to Linden Lodge?

There was a tense silence – then a quiet voice interjected from a corner of the room. It was Maureen Lingard, Head of the Junior Department. She was enormously experienced, having taught at Linden Lodge for many years, and she had the unquestioned respect of everyone: staff, parents and children alike. Her classroom was a model of calm efficiency. I'd never heard her speak loudly, let alone shout. As a young teacher, I'd often tried to figure out how she did it and even attempted to emulate her style. But it was no good – I lacked her inner tranquillity and the children could sense it.

Over the preceding months, Maureen had been fascinated to hear my anecdotes about Derek and she had said on a number of occasions how she'd love to teach him herself. Now she put her cards on the table and came up trumps as far as I was concerned. 'I'll have him in my class for a couple of terms,' she said, 'and then we can see how we go from there.'

No one could argue with that. I shot her a discreet look of gratitude across the room.

There was a further problem to solve, though: Derek's residency. When the care staff heard about the prospect of Derek boarding, more objections were raised. Where were the additional resources coming from to enable them to manage him in the evenings? How would he fit in with the other children?

I had to agree that it was far from ideal for Derek to have to come away from home for a week at a time, and commuting the forty-something miles between Wimbledon and Warfield on a daily basis wasn't a viable proposition.

Then I had a brainwave. What if Derek were to stay with Nanny in her flat in Hammersmith during the week, so that he could attend Linden Lodge as a day pupil?

This appeared to be a solution that met everyone's needs. Nanny could continue to look after Derek for a little while longer. Berkshire Education Authority would be spared the initial expense of boarding fees. And, best of all, Derek's transition to Linden Lodge would occur on a phased basis, which should keep his anxieties to a minimum.

All parties agreed to the arrangement and a date was set. Derek would attend Linden Lodge from the Monday after the autumn half-term.

At 9 a.m. prompt, the driver dropped Nanny and Derek off at the front door to North House. I was among a small welcoming party who had gathered informally to greet them. I could tell that Derek was excited – rocking so much that Nanny was barely able to keep hold of his hand. He was as immaculately turned out as ever, hair freshly shorn and a tie visible beneath his V-neck navy jumper. He listened intently to the unfamiliar voices and smelt each of the strangers' hands as he shook them.

Formalities over, I led the new boy and his chaperone through an archway in North House, round the rose beds – still there from the original Lutyens design – and over to the new building where Miss Lingard's class was to be found. Our progress was interrupted on a number of occasions by well-wishers and by the time we got to 'P2', as his new class was known, Derek had well and truly arrived at Linden Lodge. Nanny said goodbye and I escorted her to the back gate, from where it was a short walk to Southfields tube station.

'Well, there we are, Adam, it's down to Derek now.'

And Miss Lingard, I thought. I had a class waiting, so it wasn't until morning break that I could return to see how things were going. I encountered Derek en route to the playground from Maureen's room. He had evidently made a new friend – Andrew – who was helping him to find his way along the corridor. Maureen was following them discreetly. She gave me a knowing look and neither of us said anything. The boys' conversation was rather one-way, with Andrew telling Derek about the new Braille signs that he had been learning. Every now and then Derek would reply *'Yes,* Andrew', in a polite voice in which Nanny's diction was clearly discernible, though he couldn't have had an inkling of what Andrew was talking about.

So far, so good, I thought, and breathed a sigh of relief as I made my way to the staffroom for what felt like a well-deserved cup of tea.

After so much agonising over what was best for Derek, he settled into his new life without a murmur, it seemed to me. He soon got used to the regular structure of days in P2, and having Nanny in Hammersmith meant that his evenings were also secure and predictable.

I started to teach him every morning in the slot that had been recently left vacant by Philip's departure to the Midlands and the pace of his musical development quickened. Weeks passed, then months. Christmas 1986 came and went. Still his progress continued and for me an important issue was beginning to emerge. At what stage should Derek be given the opportunity to perform in public? Musically, he was already far more advanced than many of the children who regularly took part in concerts, but socially, his skills and understanding were still much more limited. However, the only way these would develop would be through direct experience. And this raised one of a number of ethical dilemmas in my mind. Was it reasonable to put Derek in the public eye without his informed consent? And wasn't there a danger that he would be demeaned by people regarding him as some kind of freak?

The answers seemed straightforward enough to me, though I knew that not everyone would agree. For example, surely it would be unfair to Derek if we *didn't* let him experience what it was like to perform in front of an audience? Had his prodigious abilities not occurred in the context of disability, he would almost certainly have been given the opportunity to celebrate his talents in a public arena by now. Therefore, if we denied Derek that chance, we would be compromising his rights as an individual – handicapping him on account of his disability. With regard to the issue of how other people viewed Derek ... to me that appeared to be a matter of taking great care with the way that he was presented: always putting Derek the person first, as 'the pianist who can't see' rather than 'the blind pianist', for instance. Indeed, it struck me that the recognition of him as a fine musician should help to promote a positive image of disabled people more generally.

The opportunity to test my arguments came sooner than I had expected. Shortly after Easter I was approached by the local Rotary Club to see whether Linden Lodge would like to put on a concert as part of a modest fund-raising event that they were organising. As the school had in the past been one of their principal beneficiaries, I was pleased to say 'yes' – it was good for the children to have the chance to do something for others. The event was to take place in Tooting Leisure Centre with a relatively small audience of around fifty people.

It seemed to be the ideal occasion for Derek's first outing as a pianist: enough of an occasion to make it a real concert, but not so significant an event that he would be exposed to the risk of humiliation should things go wrong. Nonetheless, as I had expected, there was resistance from certain quarters and I had to argue passionately for what I felt was Derek's *right*. 'We have to let him share his talents with others,' I insisted. 'Music is his life!'

In the end, it was agreed that we could go ahead, provided that the event was kept sufficiently low-profile to minimise the potential disruption to Derek's routine.

I was delighted, though also perturbed, for I hadn't confided in colleagues that a problem lay ahead to which I didn't as yet have a solution. My difficulty was this: how could I allow Derek to play freely, in his own inimitable way, while somehow keeping control of the situation? There was a real danger that in the excitement of the moment he would not stop when he got to the end of a piece, for example, but just keep going like a record stuck in the groove. Or, if the fancy took him, he might decide to perform excessively slowly or quickly, or whimsically try out a new style on the spur of the moment.

Somehow, I had to find a way of managing things unobtrusively without either having to resort to telling him what to do in front of everyone or, worse, by having to interrupt his flow through physical inter-vention. But how? I was convinced that music itself held the answer, though I couldn't immediately work out a way. Anxiously, I checked the date of the concert in my diary – Wednesday, 17 June. That gave me a little over four weeks to come up with a solution.

The phone rang. I stopped work on the song sheet that I had been brailling out and picked up the receiver.

'Someone from County Hall for you.'

It was Val, the school secretary, and without further ado she put the caller through. A quietly spoken voice on the other end of the line informed me that a school was closing down and that the assets, including, apparently, a number of pianos, were being 'redistributed' (as the man put it) on a first-come, first-served basis. He had thought of us because we had that exceptional young pianist, didn't we? (What was his name?) And, anyway, blind children liked music, didn't they?

'A lot of them do,' I replied, subtly trying to correct the stereotype without discouraging the man's genuine kindness in thinking of us. It was a fine line that I often found myself treading. The 'young pianist' he was referring to was Philip, no doubt, whose performance of the *Italian Concerto* had caught the attention of senior education officials at a London-wide youth music event in which Linden Lodge had participated. I didn't like to say that he'd left at the end of the previous academic year. Instead, I enquired how many pianos were available.

How many did I want?

I was taken aback, though I realised immediately that I shouldn't show it. Always best to give a prompt, assured answer on these occasions – and don't underestimate! 'Four,' I said, plucking a figure out of the air.

Feeling rather pleased with myself, I reported the school's latest quartet of acquisitions to Maggy Grubb. She was less than delighted, however. As far as she was concerned there was far too much clutter around the place as it was – a hangover from the Matthews era – and a fair proportion of it had something to do with music. 'What are you going to do with them, Adam?' she asked, with an undisguised testiness in her tone.

Suddenly, four sounded rather a lot. 'Well, three of them can go in the classrooms that don't currently have one,' I replied deliberately, buying myself time while mentally scouring the school for other piano-sized spaces.

Maggy's frown was fast becoming a glower.

'And . . . and we can put the spare one in the small hall for now. Good for duets,' I added rather feebly and, before she could reply, escaped to take my next lesson.

The truck that edged its way down the school's driveway first thing on Thursday morning, charting a cautious course between the day children's taxis, seemed to be unnecessarily large to accommodate four pianos, I thought. But I wasn't concerned. Perhaps we were the first of a number of deliveries.

'Have I got a surprise for you!' the driver greeted me cheerily, struggling with the stiff bolts at the back of the lorry. The doors finally swung open. 'There! What do you think of that?'

Although it was partly hidden by a number of upright pianos, shrouded in blankets, upended and held in place by means of numerous straps, there, unmistakably, was the carcass of a full-sized grand, well over six feet in length.

'County Hall thought you'd like this one too,' he said, giving the near end a friendly slap.

My mouth opened to say something, then closed again in a mixture of astonishment and horror.

The man only read the surprise in my face, though, and he laughed. 'Glad to see you're pleased.'

A vision of an irate Maggy started to swim before my eyes. We were close friends as well as colleagues, and she was among the most kind-hearted people I knew, but fools, suffer and gladly were not three concepts that were readily juxtaposed in her mind.

'Hope you've got a lot of space. It's huge!' He chuckled again.

'Let's go round the back,' I said, quickly thinking what to do. 'It'll be easier to unload from there.'

The four uprights were dispatched to their various locations with relative ease. That left the grand.

'Through here.' I darted a nervous glance around the entrance hall and up towards the staffroom as I held the doors to the gym wide open. I wanted to tell the two men to be as quick as they could, but pushing the body of the heavy piano, strapped sideways on to a special trolley, up the sloping corridor from the back entrance of the building was not something to be rushed. And, after all, this was the fifth instrument they'd moved that morning. My concern was that the bell was about to go for morning break and I knew Maggy was on duty.

The men negotiated the turn into the gym.

I breathed a sigh of relief and closed the doors behind them. We still had to get it out of sight, though.

'Whereabouts d'you want it, mate?' the older of the two men asked.

I looked at him awkwardly. 'Sorry about this, but up on the stage, please.'

There was a pause, then a brief interchange during which it was established that I wasn't, in fact, joking. I offered to help, but health and safety rules wouldn't permit it. So I went to get two cups of tea, instead, four sugars in each, as instructed.

When I returned a few minutes later, I was relieved to see that the men were already on the stage, starting to put the piano back on its legs. Then the bell went. Quickly, I put the teas down on the apron, jumped up into the wings and closed the curtains.

'Now what are you doing?' asked the younger man.

'Er . . . I want it to be a surprise,' I said, feeling myself becoming tangled in a Basil Fawlty-like web.

I just had time to see the piano movers off before the bell went again for the end of break and to signal to the juniors that they should gather in the small hall for one of their thrice-weekly singing lessons with me. If an inspector had asked why it was necessary to have three of these get-togethers every five days, Maureen Lingard would no doubt have pointed to the value of the sessions as an opportunity for all the younger pupils to engage in a common pursuit. It was particularly difficult to find activities in which a group of thirty or so visually impaired children, with a wide range of abilities and other disabilities, could purposefully participate at the same time. I did wonder whether the class teachers' desire for 'free periods' was also a factor in their unreservedly positive view of music lessons. I had no objection, though, since working with all the children together was an efficient way of teaching them a repertoire that subsequently served as a source of material for more creative work in individual and class lessons.

I got a few of the first-comers to set out the chairs as I lined up our new piano with the old one – two Danemanns side by side. Apart from some differences in wear and tear on their cases they looked very much the same, and I wondered how many such instruments the Inner London Education Authority must have purchased over the years. Seeing them there together gave me an idea, and when Derek came in, last as ever, I took him by the hand and led him to one of the piano stools.

'Good news, everyone,' I announced. 'We've got *two* pianos in the small hall today.' I put my hand on Derek's shoulder. 'And I've got someone to help me play the accompaniment.'

'Derek!' called out a couple of the children who could see enough to know.

He grinned and clapped his hands together in delight.

'Now, who would like to choose the first song?'

As usual, a forest of arms shot up.

'Mmm, let's see . . .' Out of the corner of my eye I saw Maureen walking past the door to the hall.

'Who's sitting up the straightest?' I could play the schoolteacher when I had to, though it didn't come naturally.

My attention was drawn to a little girl in the front row who was evidently trying with all her might to sit up straight and still, though she couldn't stop her fingers and wrists flapping with excitement. In one hand she was holding aloft a rather battered home-made spiral-bound book, which had clearly seen better days, fluttering like a hopeful flag, eager to be chosen. There was a small bell on the cover that was jangling as she waved the book. I couldn't resist: 'Claire, what would you like?'

With desperate eagerness she thumbed through the sheets of card, rubbing the fingers of her right hand over the small objects that were stuck to the pages – a different one on each. There was a little square of sponge, a typewriter key, a small plastic star, a metal ring and many others. After some deliberation she chose the page with a plastic peg and handed me the open book. On it was the music to 'Everyday' – the Buddy Holly classic.

'"Everyday", Claire, is that right?' I asked, partly to check that I had understood correctly and partly to let the children who hadn't been able to follow proceedings visually know what she had chosen.

Claire vocalised back, affirming her choice. She wasn't able to speak and her fingers weren't sensitive enough to read Braille. She was passionate about music, though, and her frustration at being unable to choose the pieces that *she* wanted had in the past resulted in her becoming increasingly self-destructive. Only a few months previously she would often scream with rage and bang her head repeatedly. It was agonising to watch her becoming so upset, but sometimes, the more one tried to help, the worse matters became as misunderstanding degenerated into ever deeper confusion.

Something had had to be done and I had begun

by making Claire a tactile songbook. Each page had a small object attached to it that she could identify and which for her symbolised a different song. The corresponding music was copied on to the page so that whoever was taking the music lesson could play it for her. Rarely, in teaching, did simple ideas like this result in a breakthrough: usually small improvements would come about after years of patient engagement with a child. But on this occasion the results were truly dramatic and, within only a few weeks, Claire was able to choose from twenty of her favourite songs.

I had only got as far as the first 'tick' of the introduction to 'Everyday' when, without being prompted, Derek joined in on his piano with a replica of the clock that I habitually created in sound at the beginning of the song. As ever, I was amused, humbled and, above all, enchanted to watch his fingers effortlessly finding the right keys and through their actions intrigued to imagine his mind at work. Derek had heard me play the piece many times before, of course, as I had taught the juniors the song over a number of sessions, but I'd never noticed him playing it before. That was one of the odd things about Derek, as Nanny had observed years earlier. In order to learn a piece, he didn't physically have to practise it or even play it through. All he had to do was just listen a few times and it would be there, ready and waiting, for whenever he wanted to call it up – sometimes years later.

Working with a large group of children who couldn't see their teacher presented a number of challenges for both parties. Clearly, conducting was out of the question, so starting and stopping, slowing down and speeding up, and making expressive changes or effects such as getting louder or softer had to be co-ordinated non-visually: through sound, using speech or musical cues. As I soon discovered, calling out what was required was disruptive and in any case spoken instructions meant little to several of the children (including Derek). So, during a performance, the direction of the group had to come solely through inflections in the piano part, to which the children learnt to listen very attentively. For example, if a verse were to be sung sadly, then the accompaniment might reflect this through a reduction in tempo and dynamics and, perhaps, by moving to the 'minor' key. Conversely, the return to a happy state could be conveyed through an increase in movement, loudness and the use of 'major' chords. It was even possible to communicate a sense of irony, which could be appreciated by some of the older and more able pupils, by juxtaposing different pieces with contrasting connotations together – for example, by playing fragments of 'Day-oh!' while the children were singing 'Morning Has Broken'.

The accompaniment could relay simpler messages too. For instance, if a chorus were to be repeated at the end, this could be signalled through particular chords that suggested there was more to come. From time to time I would link songs together by improvising a 'bridge' between them. Musically, this would borrow material from the first piece and incrementally transform it into the introduction to the second, so it gradually became apparent what this was to be. Sometimes the children would compete to see who could name the upcoming tune first. If things were becoming too straightforward, I would tease them by appearing to set off in a certain direction, only to change course at the last moment. Increasingly, I was able to hold their attention by linking a whole sequence of pieces in this way. Indeed, I came to the conclusion that the most effective lessons were those in which there was little or no talking, and that the more one could teach music *through* music the better.

Hearing Derek imitate my introduction to 'Everyday' and sensing the feeling of anticipation among the group, the temptation to explore the new possibilities that his presence at the keyboard offered was irresistible. I started by keeping the clock going longer than usual: maintaining the repeated rhythm of the 'ticks' but progressively introducing different chords that didn't yet allow the children to start singing the tune. Immediately, Derek was with me – following the pattern of harmonies that I established and improvising more 'ticks' and 'tocks' up the chromatic scale. I couldn't resist the workings of the clock becoming even more exotic, and diminished chords were replaced by whole-tone clusters. Then, with the ticking continuing all the time, I introduced fragments from 'The Rhythm of Life' which Derek took up with alacrity. Once the rhythm was pulsating in everyone's fingers and feet, I led the music back, step by step, to the late 1950s and a style with which Buddy Holly would hopefully have felt some

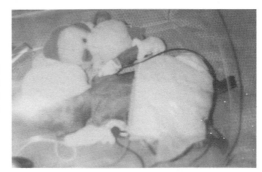

Weighing little more than 700g, newborn Derek fights for life in an incubator.

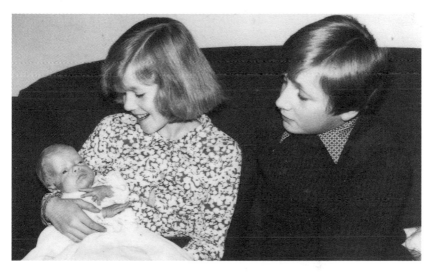

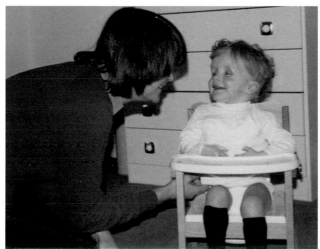

Home at last with Libbet and Charles, October 1979.

Sharing a joke with Mary Ann (aged 1).

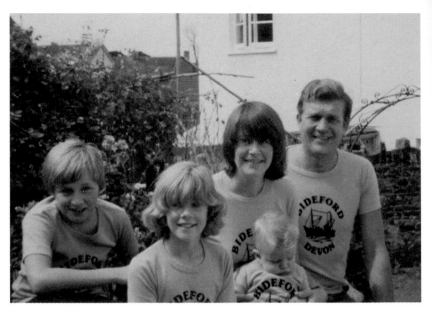

The Paravicini family on holiday in Bideford, August 1980.

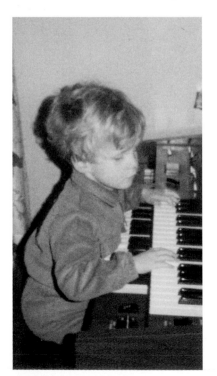

Playing Nic's Yamaha, aged 3.

Holding on tight to Nanny,
in Guernsey, 1983.

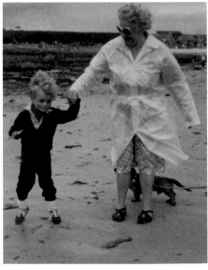

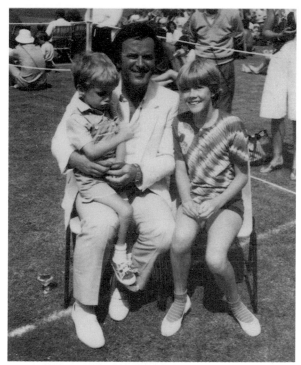

Derek's *first* meeting with Terry Wogan, aged 4.

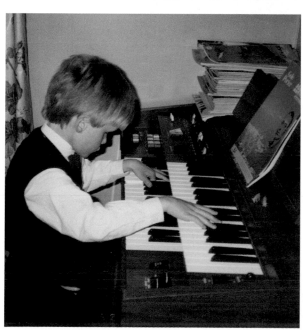

Playing both manuals on the organ (1985).

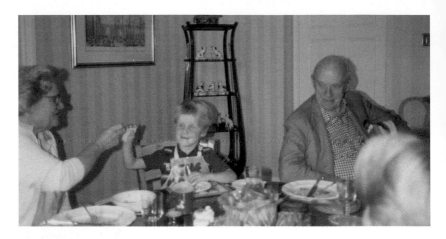

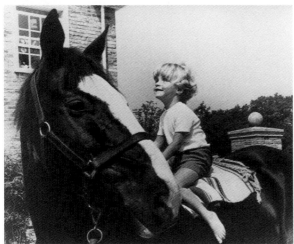

'Cheers', with Nanny and Uncle John (Lord Glendevon) in Guernsey, aged 5.

'Two great survivors'. Derek and Sefton at North Lodge Farm.

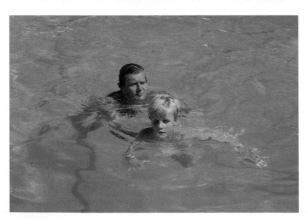

Swimming with Nic in 1985.

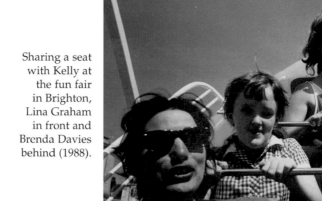

Sharing a seat with Kelly at the fun fair in Brighton, Lina Graham in front and Brenda Davies behind (1988).

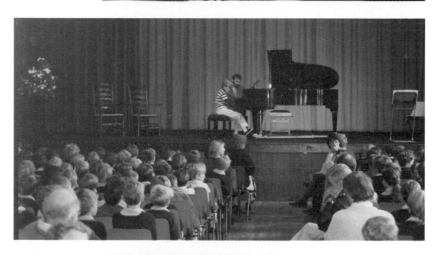

Entertaining pupils at the Dragon School, Oxford, in 1990.

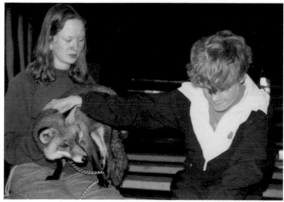

Getting to grips with nature at a wildlife park in Hertfordshire, 1994.

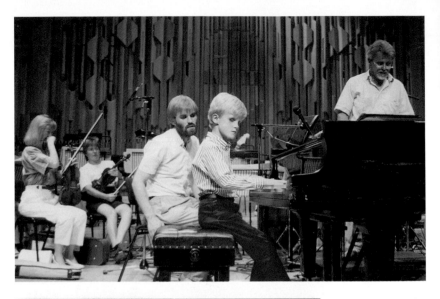

Trying out the
piano at the
Barbican with
the Philharmonic
(aged 9).

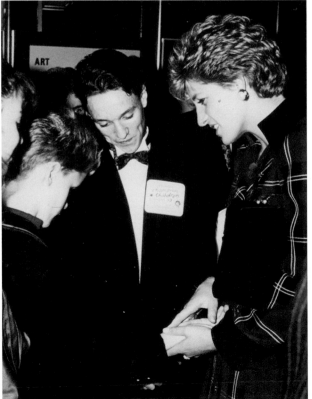

Diana meets
Derek (aged 14),
wart and all.

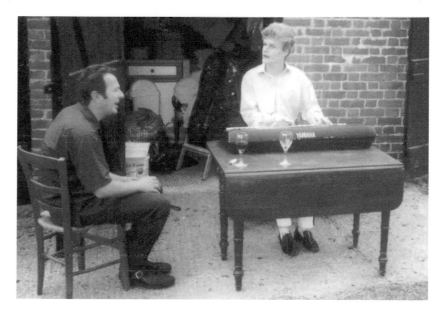

Strumming with Joe
in the late '90s.

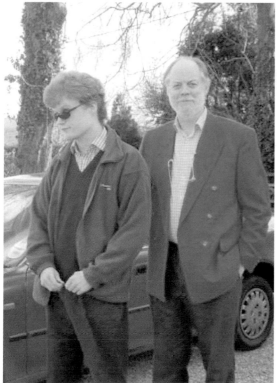

Off to a concert
with John Lubbock,
conductor of the
Orchestra of St John's,
2003. © Antony Hanbury

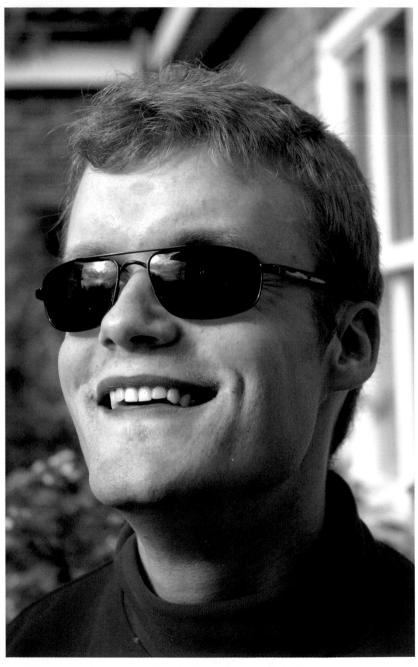

Taking a break from recording his first CD at the RNIB Soundscape Centre, Surrey, 2005. © 2005, Evangelos Himonides affinity. Finally we played the chord that the children had been waiting for, and they knew just when to come in.

And then it dawned on me. Here was the solution to the problem of keeping Derek's playing within bounds during public performance. He would have one (the main) keyboard while I would discreetly accompany him on another, allowing him as much freedom as possible, but ultimately having control as to what style and tempo pieces should be played in and, if necessary, determining when they should end. 'Everyday' had shown that Derek was now prepared to follow me, but not slavishly: we could have a genuine musical dialogue in which he was the more prominent voice, but in which I was ultimately the senior partner. It felt rather like walking along with a young child, where the adult keeps a steady pace and a sense of the overall direction, while the infant runs this way and that with an air of youthful excitement, but returning periodically to the security of the carer.

'Everyday' was coming to an end but I wanted the musical magic to continue, so I decided to segue into 'Every Night' an old Appalachian folksong with similarities to the Blues. The clock wound down and its regular 'tick' was replaced by a gentle swing rhythm. This time I left Derek to introduce the tune. He did, and the children followed.

So, one problem solved, I thought, pleased with myself – a good morning's work. Then I remembered the grand piano. What should I do about that? I half turned to watch Derek, who had now added a full rock 'n' roll accompaniment to 'Every Night'. There was only one answer. I resolved to take the bull by the horns and have him play for the whole school on the new instrument during assembly the next day. I would accompany him for the hymns on the upright. That way there would be two new things for people to contemplate at the same time. And hopefully, Maggy would be so pleased with Derek's music-making that her mind would be taken off the fact that most of the stage was now taken up with more of my 'clutter'.

As it turned out, I was correct in my first assumption but not in the second. But all dust settles in the end.

Nanny, ever a willing draftee, was called upon to assist on the evening of the concert and to represent the family, as Nic and Mary Ann were away. She joined the small gaggle of children clustered around Maureen Lingard and two other staff at the side entrance to North House, waiting for me to unlock the minibus. There too were Nicky and Hayley, girls three years older than Derek, both fine singers with an unusual maturity of vocal production. Hayley, in particular, had a rich vibrato and a haunting tonal quality that within two years was to be heard in the Royal Albert Hall and on television. Fiona, slightly younger than Derek, was clutching a descant recorder in one hand and a guitar in the other. Three other juniors, Kelly (the girl Derek had pushed off the piano stool the day I met him), Joanne and Neil, had also come along, completing a respectable vocal group of seven, capable of singing rounds and part songs, as well as backing some of the popular numbers that Nicky and Hayley were to perform.

Nanny was in her element, immensely proud of Derek and delighted to be with him on his first public musical outing, aged just seven years and eleven months. Derek could sense the feeling of anticipation in the air and he was excited too, rocking back and forth as ever, despite Nanny's secure grip on his wrist.

The twelve of us packed ourselves into the minibus around the two keyboards, amplifier, microphones, leads and a small mixer that I had loaded earlier, and, all aboard, we made our way through the rush hour traffic to Tooting. The worst part of these events was having to move the gear around, which was at once heavy, awkward and fragile.

I was still setting up and checking the balance of the microphones at the leisure centre as the audience began to drift in: mainly parents, friends and the Rotarians who had organised the concert. The children who were going to perform sat to one side with Maureen, Nanny and the two helpers.

I'd organised the programme so that Derek was on third after an introductory song by Hayley and a spot by Fiona that involved her playing the recorder and accompanying her own singing on the guitar. That way I reckoned that he would have time enough to get used to the atmosphere without having to wait too long for his turn.

After the applause had died down following

Fiona's vocal and instrumental version of 'Blowing in the Wind', I led her back to her chair.

'Your turn, Derek,' I said, taking him by the hand and leading him to the larger of the two keyboards, which was nearer the audience. Maureen had agreed to announce the piece so that I could be ready to start things off with an introduction that would set the appropriate mood and tempo before Derek had time to jump in with whatever was in his head at the time.

'Good evening, Ladies and Gentlemen,' she said in her softly spoken but authoritative way. 'I would now like to introduce Derek Paravicini, who is performing in public for the first time tonight.'

I glanced at Nanny. I could see that she, like me, was listening to Maureen, but her eyes were on Derek, willing him to do well. He was rocking slowly on the piano stool, his fingers fidgeting in readiness for their forthcoming workout. He smiled when he heard his name and sat still for a moment to give his full attention to what Miss Lingard was saying.

'He's going to play the "Streets of London".'

Derek's smile widened into a broad beam that stretched right across his face. This was the moment that he'd been waiting for.

I decided to assert my authority straight away – and to keep Derek on his toes – by beginning in E flat major, a key in which he had not, as far as I could remember, ever played the song. I couldn't think of another child (except, perhaps, Philip) for whom such an act wouldn't have had disastrous consequences. But for Derek, the unusual was commonplace and I had complete faith in his ability to follow me. My confidence was well-founded and before the opening chord had faded away he was there alongside me, as though it were the most natural thing in the world to play a piece in an unfamiliar key before his first ever public audience. The hundreds of hours that we had spent practising all conceivable scales and arpeggios had refined his raw capacity to realise his entire repertoire starting on any note, and he was now equally at home playing pieces in any key – rather like being able to speak twelve languages with native fluency.

I led Derek resolutely through the first verse and chorus of the 'Streets of London' and he obediently followed. I was longing to let him go in order to see just where his musical imagination, fired up by the excitement of the occasion, would take us, and as soon as I judged it was prudent to do so – towards the end of verse two – I gradually retreated into the background with a series of *sotto voce* chords. The instant that he sensed my musical grip was released, Derek was off, scampering up the octave with a series of broken chords. Up and up he took the music, ascending into higher and higher realms of musical invention. Just when it seemed as though he was going to run out of notes at the end of the keyboard, he came scurrying down in a series of tumbling scales and rejoined me in the middle register. Seizing my opportunity, I took the lead again and introduced a new syncopated rhythm in the bass. Without a moment's hesitation his left hand too started skipping along to the new beat before he broke free once more, dancing out of my reach.

And so our *pas de deux* continued for a few minutes, until it felt appropriate to draw matters to a close, before Derek ran out of steam and his perambulations became repetitive. An almost imperceptible reduction in the pace of my accompaniment signalled that it was time to wind things up, and he fell back into step with a series of expansive chords that served as an effective climax to the piece. He held on the last fortissimo cluster of notes, waiting for me to lift my hands up first, then he couldn't resist his trademark final plonk low down in the left hand.

The audience burst into rapturous applause – this was quite unlike anything they'd ever seen or heard before. There were shouts of 'Well done, Derek!' He was quivering with excitement, his face radiant, his hands alternately clapping and flapping energetically at his sides. I looked across at Nanny. She too was applauding vigorously, her eyes shining with pride. I felt relieved, delighted and (I had to admit) vindicated. From somewhere, Derek seemed to have acquired the instincts of a natural performer: a sense of occasion and the capacity to rise to it, the ability to communicate with an audience and a feeling of exhilaration when his playing was acknowledged. These were things that could not be taught, but with them, Derek's playing had the potential to reach heights that were as yet unexplored.

'D'you think she'd ever agree?' Maureen looked up from the list of names with a quizzical smile on her face.

'I think she'd be all right about it with you and me there, Maureen. If we promise to look after him carefully!'

I was sure that Derek would have a great time and it was the obvious next step to take. We were planning the annual school trip to the Woodlarks campsite in Surrey. In previous years this had been the preserve of the younger seniors, but it had been decided that this summer the juniors should go, and Maureen was preparing to write to parents of the day children to see how many would allow them to go away for the week.

As far as Derek was concerned, we decided that it would be best if I sounded out Nanny first and, somewhat to my surprise, she immediately saw the benefits for Derek in what we were proposing. 'I'm sure he'll have a lovely time, Adam. Now, I wonder if he's got all the things he'll need.'

When Nanny did something, she did it properly, and I could imagine Derek turning up complete with a tent, Primus stove, mess kit, fold-down chair and provisions for the week.

'Don't worry Nanny – everything will be there waiting for us.' And I explained about the Woodlarks site, which specialised in offering people with disabilities a taste of the outdoors. Large tents were provided and there was a cookhouse with a wood-burning range. There were also washrooms, toilets and a laundry and – more interesting as far as the children were concerned – an outdoor heated swimming pool, set in the middle of the woods. It was an idyllic spot and I'd seen even the most tense of children gradually unwind over the week as they settled into the relaxed pace of life, away from the relentless routine of the classroom.

As I anticipated, Derek was no exception. It was a glorious sunny week and he was perfectly happy, sitting or lying on a rug outside his tent, soaking up the sun like a lizard – though one whose head was constantly on the move, rocking this way or that. As a result, he developed a beautifully even tan, his skin golden brown and his hair fairer than ever.

Derek loved the facilities that Woodlarks had to offer. He was fearless in the water and was quite happy to be thrown in the deep end, bobbing back to the surface each time like a cork. He enjoyed exploring in the woods, feeling the crack of twigs underfoot, taking in the scent of the moist leaf mould that was released, hearing the wind rustling the leaves of the trees overhead and listening to the birds calling to one another from near and far. He took great delight in the after-supper singing round the campfire, joining in lustily. It constantly amazed me how quickly many of the children could learn not only the music of songs but the words too – even when many of the lyrics couldn't have made much sense to them.

With Derek, the disparity between the very limited language that he was able to understand and deploy in everyday situations and his enormous repertoire of song and hymn texts was particularly striking. Nanny had discovered quite early on that he could also learn swathes of poetry with seemingly little effort – all beautifully enunciated, in emulation of her – but apparently with no comprehension at all. Nanny and I had discussed this at some length in the past. It was the equivalent, we decided, of our remembering long tracts in a foreign language, of which the occasional word might be recognisable but which, on the whole, was unintelligible. There was no doubt that we would find it very difficult indeed. So how was Derek able to accomplish this seemingly impossible feat? For him, we decided, poetry was just another series of rhythmically inflected sounds, which he could learn in the same way that he was able to assimilate music, through a sophisticated process of pattern identification, storage and retrieval. It was all sustenance for his eclectic and insatiable appetite for sound.

Woodlarks even had a piano – of sorts. It was kept in a large barn, which served admirably as an indoor dining and leisure area in wet weather, but offered little protection against the damp or the cold in winter. As a consequence, a number of the piano's notes had ceased to function altogether and joined the choir inaudible, as I thought of it, and those that survived were so out of tune that they sounded like an ill-tempered gamelan. Yet, miraculously, Derek was somehow able to breathe a beauteous order into the clangorous beastie: his fingers raced around more than usual, seeking out the notes that worked best and had the truest intonation. For the final night, the piano was wheeled outside as far as it would go on the hard-standing beyond the cookhouse, and with Derek taking requests, everyone gathered round in a circle and sang till they were hoarse.

Finally, the children wended their way to their tents for the last time (some of them managing rather better in the dark than the staff!) and I found myself walking beside Maureen, who, torch in hand, was helping Derek to get his bearings. He was as full of life as ever, buzzing with the excitement of the evening, but relaxed and smiling.

'Thanks for a great week, Miss Lingard,' I said, Nanny-like, trying to verbalise what he might be thinking. Then directly to him: 'You've had good time, haven't you, Derek?'

'You *have*, Adam,' he said emphatically, his grasp of pronouns as hazy as ever.

But the sentiment was unequivocal.

The following September there were a number of changes at Linden Lodge, brought about by the shifting population of visually impaired children that we served. There were now so many pupils in the junior school – due in part to the large increase in the number of babies who, like Derek, had been surviving in recent years with *retinopathy of prematurity* – that an additional class was needed for eight- and nine-year-olds. Maggy Grubb had approached me in July to see whether I would be interested in taking on such a group. She expected there to be six boys, five of whom were at various stages of learning Braille, and one who used large print. Having to get to grips with the primary curriculum would be a whole new challenge for me, which would undoubtedly absorb most of the summer holidays, though the prospect of working with six lively and open young minds for a year was very appealing. However, becoming a class teacher would inevitably mean a reduction in the time I had available to teach music. It was a hard choice, but in the end I decided to take the opportunity for the added experience it would bring.

Although, in terms of age, Derek would have been a natural candidate for my new class, the extent of his learning difficulties meant that he needed a more experiential programme than I was able to offer. As a result, it was decided that he should transfer instead to Lina Graham's class for children who had special needs in addition to their sight problems. Claire, the girl for whom I had made a tactile song-book, was there, as was Kelly, who had sung at the concert in Tooting. Brand had just joined too. Like so many of the other children, he had a fine musical ear including 'perfect pitch': for him, each note was distinctive. However, his hemiplegia meant that it was very difficult for him to use his right hand, though he was able to play the piano quite effect-ively using his left alone.

The final member of the class was Thabo, who, with his sister, had been subject to dreadful physical abuse as a baby. He alone had survived, somehow, though he was left blind and severely brain-damaged. The prospects for any real quality of life seemed bleak. What was there that he would enjoy, that would bring him out of himself and back into the world of other people? It turned out that music – especially pieces with a strong rhythm – would kick-start him into action. When the juniors sang

'Rockin' All over the World' full blast, with Derek and me giving the two pianos hell, it ignited Thabo and his whole being would see-saw along to the beat in a state of great excitement. He just loved it. And, best of all, rhythm provided a secure and predictable framework that encouraged and supported the development of his speech.

So music was important, in one way or another, for each individual in Lina's class and a special chemistry existed between the children, in which music was the catalyst for social interaction. Their differing abilities and needs complemented each other perfectly and, unlikely as it seemed, the five of them were capable of functioning as an autonomous musical group. Derek and Brand played the keyboards, Thabo was on percussion (the congas were his favourite) and Kelly and Claire led on the vocals. One or other of the girls also took the lead in determining which piece should be performed next, since decision-making was not the boys' strong suit.

Lina and I were as different as the proverbial chalk and cheese. She had trained as a specialist to teach children with learning difficulties and for her music was largely of value as a means to an end in promoting wider development. She was quiet and unassuming, and the children instinctively liked and trusted her. I quickly came to the conclusion that she wasn't instinctively a performer and she found it difficult to see why putting children with Derek's level of disability in the public eye could possibly be of any benefit to them at all. Which was a shame, because in mid September the Rotary Club got back to me and asked whether Linden Lodge would consider putting on a much larger concert at Wandsworth Town Hall – this time in front of several hundred people.

Sensing a battle ahead, I marshalled the arguments I had used before, but this time with the added advantage that Derek had one concert under his belt and no one who had seen him in action could deny his obvious pleasure in interacting with an audience. In the end, Lina had to agree, though I had the feeling that Derek and I were both on probation in her mind.

As it was a much bigger event, I decided to involve the seniors too, and Hayley, Nicky, Derek and the rest were joined by a number of older performers, including Terry on the drums, Peter on the synthesiser and Carlo on vocals. The music ranged from ragtime to reggae and rapping to rock. Derek played duets with me as he had done previously, this time performing on the Town Hall's grand piano while I accompanied on an electric keyboard. We changed places to back the girls' singing and, for the first time, Derek was able to function as part of a group that included drums and guitar. I'd noticed in rehearsal that he had a tendency to play everyone's parts, not just his own, which at first had seemed both amazing and amusing. However, I just couldn't find a way of getting across to him that there was no need to double the vocal line, the lead guitar and the bass, so humour quickly gave way to bemusement as I struggled to involve Derek without him dominating the group. In the end, it came down to my judicious use of the volume control on his keyboard – though we'd hit upon a problem that was to colour Derek's ensemble playing for years to come.

The evening was hailed as a great success. Derek's extended family turned out in force to see his first significant public appearance, demonstrating a loyalty to him and an enthusiasm for his achievements that continues to this day. They could never have imagined that the tiny baby they had first seen at North Lodge Farm would ever achieve so much. Mary Ann in particular was convinced that his feisty, spirited playing was somehow a reflection of his early fight for life. It felt as though Derek, aged eight, had really *arrived* at last. Severely disabled he might be, but through his music he now had developed a personal identity to which they could all relate. Of course, neither they nor I could have dreamt at the time that what we had just witnessed was only the beginning of Derek's remarkable achievements. But the next step had already been envisaged by one person in the audience, upon whom Derek's playing had left a deep impression. This chance encounter, of which we were wholly unaware, was shortly to have a profound influence on the course of Derek's life.

Chapter Five

In the Public Eye

'Adam. *Adam!*' Maggy's voice rang out as she walked down the corridor towards the small hall. 'Will you get the men to sort these cables out, *now!*'

'Sorry,' I said quietly to Lucy Pilkington, with whom I'd been discussing how to handle things after break. 'I'd better go and see what's up.'

I pushed open the door from the hall and peered into the lobby where three corridors and a flight of stairs leading up to the first floor all converged. Lina's classroom and a cloakroom lay just beyond. But all these familiar features passed me by as I momentarily froze with horror at the sight that met my eyes. Where a quarter of an hour before there had been a clear walkway, the floor was now scarcely visible beneath coils of thick grey cables, some of which were connected to large lights on stands, while others disappeared towards electrical sockets up the corridor where Maggy was standing. One even snaked its way out of an open window. Worst of all, a particularly large light was half blocking the entrance to Lina's classroom. On hearing Maggy's voice she too had put her head round the door, and she glared at me tight-lipped. 'You *promised* us there would be no disruption. The children wouldn't even notice what was going on, you said. And now look at this. It'll be break time in a couple of minutes.'

She was right to be concerned. Very soon, twenty or so pairs of unseeing feet would be at a high risk of becoming ensnared in the tangle of wires. The men who had left them there had temporarily disappeared and we couldn't hope to shift them all ourselves before the bell went.

I could think of only one thing to do. Take up position on point duty. But Maggy, practical as ever, was ahead of me – already directing Lina and Lucy to strategic locations around the web and stationing herself by the stairs, ready to warn children to wait for help. I moved to the middle of the circle of cables and stood, rather like a benign spider, ready to assist them in getting across. They would need to be particularly careful to avoid the lights that were enmeshed in the wires like giant stick insects.

Needless to say, when they arrived, the children weren't fazed at all – indeed, many of them were fascinated to feel just how thick the cables were and track them up the corridor, to get some idea of the dimensions of the lights perched on their large metallic stands and to manipulate the shutters to see how they worked. It reminded me of the situation a few months before when, following the infamous hurricane that had struck the south of England, a number of large trees had been uprooted in and around the school grounds: a natural calamity, for sure, but one which presented a unique learning opportunity for children with no sight. Until then their experience of a tree had for the most part been limited to feeling around the trunk, perhaps grabbing at low-hanging twigs and leaves, or even scrambling a short way up on the bottom branches. Now, though, with entire specimens horizontal on the ground they could get some idea of their height, appreciate the sheer scale of their crowns and explore the gnarling complexity of their root systems. There is no substitute for hands-on experiences like these to build up concepts of things that sighted people generally take for granted.

For the moment, though, surrounded by a growing crowd of increasingly excited children outside the small hall, Maggy was more concerned with health and safety issues than the opportunities to learn about filming on location. 'Come on, keep moving,' she ordered. 'If you're interested, Adam can show you everything in small groups during lunch break.'

So much for my trip to the pub with Lucy and the crew, then. But I could hardly complain, given the chaos I was causing.

It had all started a month or so previously when I'd had a call from a researcher on the *People* programme, which was to be screened by the BBC in the summer. It was hosted by Derek Jameson, a rumbustious character, who put himself across as having the common touch and a heart of gold. Each half-hour slot profiled three or four hitherto unknown personalities who were judged to be particularly interesting, on account of their unusual hobbies, habits, exploits or expertise. By chance, a contact had seen Derek's recent performance at Wandsworth Town Hall and she had thought that he might be a suitable candidate for the show.

A number of conflicting thoughts swirled through my mind as the researcher described what participation in the programme would be likely to entail – at least a couple of days filming at Linden Lodge to illustrate Derek's musical talents and to give some impression of what he was like as a person. How would he react to being filmed, the young woman wanted to know. What would his parents feel about it? Would the school be amenable to the idea? These were questions that I simply couldn't answer there and then, so I stalled, saying that I would have to give the matter some thought. In the meantime I agreed to meet Lucy Pilkington, one of the co-presenters on the programme, to talk things through and allow her to meet Derek.

I pondered the proposal fitfully during a restless night in my room in North House. First of all, before contemplating other people's views, I tried as far as possible to think on behalf of Derek. In this context, had he been able to understand, what would *he* have thought? I had to admit that the proposition sounded both exciting and hazardous at the same time. It was a difficult judgement to make, particularly since I sensed that a huge amount potentially hung on it – in principle, the whole of Derek's future direction as a performer. If his talents really were to be given the public attention that I felt they deserved, this type of media exposure was inevitable. So we would have to bite the bullet sooner or later. But was now the right time? Shouldn't we wait until he was older when, perhaps, he would have developed some understanding of what the process of filming and broadcasting meant, and therefore could make more of an informed decision for himself? But how long would that be? (Indeed, would he *ever* develop that level of comprehension? There was no way of knowing.) In any case, another opportunity to appear on national television might not come along for some time – if at all.

It became clear that this line of reasoning had too many imponderables and was leading nowhere. So I tried a different tack – asking myself questions that were more readily answerable. First, what would Derek be likely to get out of the experience? The main argument I had used for him performing in concerts – that he relished the opportunity for social interaction which such events offered – didn't really hold water, since there wouldn't be a live audience with whom he could engage. Second, what could go wrong? The main risk appeared to lie in Derek's unpredictable behaviour, and as we wouldn't have any editorial control over the piece that went out – what was included and the way in which he was portrayed – there was a fair chance that he would be misrepresented.

So that was that. The response to Lucy and the team had to be 'no', since the potential costs outweighed the possible benefits. With that thought, I finally managed to get off to sleep.

But it wasn't long before I was awake again, stirred by a nagging doubt. Surely this *couldn't* be the correct decision. It was Derek's right to enjoy the same opportunities and to take the same risks as everyone else, and who was I to deny him the chance of a lifetime? I got out of bed, turned on the light, sat at my desk and attempted to draft some ground rules that could be used to inform his participation in the *People* programme – or, indeed, in any similar event in the future. I couldn't bear to go through this mental anguish again: the issue needed sorting out once and for all.

The first principle I came up with was that Derek should be encouraged and supported to make an informed choice as far as he possibly could. Second, where Derek was not able to make a decision for himself, his teachers or carers and family should come to a view on his behalf that they believed to be in his best interests. Third, whatever the activity entailed it should be an enjoyable experience for Derek. Fourth, any depiction or description of Derek should be fair and accurate, celebrating his achievements, certainly, but without either demeaning him (through having him perform 'circus tricks', for example) or senti-mentalising his 'triumph over adversity'.

It occurred to me, though, that these principles represented only half the picture: our obligations to Derek. What could reasonably be expected of him? I felt strongly that he should be taught to take on certain responsibilities too. For example, if he agreed to play in a concert or take part in a produc-tion, then beyond a certain point in time, he needed to appreciate that it wouldn't be acceptable for him to pull out, since that would mean letting down an audience and, perhaps, fellow performers. Similarly, out of respect for those who were listening to him or playing along with him, he should always strive to give of his best.

In the cold light of day this ethical framework still seemed to me to strike the right balance, and it proved to be a useful focus for discussion with Derek's family and my colleagues at Linden Lodge. A consensus soon emerged that it would be appropriate for him to take part in the programme. Now it was up to me to make sure that all went well.

It took the rest of the morning for the team from the BBC to fix up the lights in the small hall, agree the camera positions and to rehearse what was going to happen. I had made it clear to them that they would only get one attempt to film the sequence they wanted. I couldn't guarantee Derek's co-operation beyond that. In any case, as I'd said to Lucy, I didn't expect things to pan out the way they were hoping, but she'd urged me to 'give it a go' . . . 'Don't worry, Adam, if it doesn't work out, it doesn't work out, and all we'll have lost is an hour of time and a few reels of tape.'

What they were hoping to capture was Derek's supposed power of 'instant recall': the ability to listen to a piece of music once and then play it straight back flawlessly. Belief in this capacity has been at the core of musical savant folklore ever since the publication of Mark Twain's account of 'Blind Tom' in the second half of the nineteenth century. I have an abiding suspicion of the accuracy of such tales of people's 'photographic memory' for sound, however. How would the audience have known whether the reproduction had been truly accurate or not? And in whose interests would it have been to say that the feat had been less than perfectly accomplished? The story wouldn't have been nearly as compelling.

The whole issue had recently been reinforced by the first appearance on television of the young autistic artist Stephen Wiltshire in the BBC programme *The Foolish Wise Ones*. He had drawn a detailed pencil sketch of the Victorian Gothic façade of St Pancras railway station in London after looking at it for only a few moments. If Stephen could manage that, Lucy had suggested, then presumably Derek could do the same in music?

'No,' I'd stated firmly. 'That's not how his mind works.'

I'd tried to explain that he did indeed have a remarkable memory, but that it operated over the *long term*. He learnt pieces by listening to them several times over (just how many hearings were necessary depended on the length and complexity of the piece), after which he seemed to have a faithful and permanent record of them. But what he *didn't* have the capacity to do was to play back several minutes' worth of complicated music immediately after he'd heard it. Relatively straightforward pieces with plenty of repetition (pop songs, for example) were a different matter: Derek could usually get the gist of those very quickly. And he had the unusual facility for playing along with an unfamiliar piece – at least, that's what he seemed to be doing. In fact, if you listened carefully, you'd notice that he was a fraction of a second behind the performance that he was hearing. He was able to do this since his musical reactions were so incredibly quick. But neither of these things was equivalent to Stephen's 'eidetic' memory, in which visual images were stored camera-like: swiftly and in breathtaking detail.

In reality, as my work with Derek and the psychologist Professor Linda Pring has subsequently shown, his memory functions much more like a 'sonic jigsaw puzzle solver' than a tape recorder. The first time he hears unfamiliar music, he remembers features and fragments of it, rather like the pieces of a jigsaw in sound. He also retains a good idea of its overall size and shape. But as he reconstructs the music (when he is asked to play it back), the musical chunks that he can remember are quite likely to appear in the wrong order.

So how does he make it all work?

In Derek's brain there appears to be a veritable 'music factory', capable of tailoring or producing new melodic or harmonic fragments on demand that fit in precisely with the needs of the moment. Not only that, but he seems to have access to a library of thousands (perhaps millions) of musical 'jigsaw pieces' that he has heard before, from which he can instantly select those that are appropriate for a given 'puzzle' in which there are gaps.

The result is that whatever Derek comes up with always makes, at the very least, good musical sense.

Occasionally, though, he manages to recreate music after a first hearing that is both striking and memorable, bearing some resemblances to the original, though never a simple replica of it. Give him time to mull over the music, however, away from the piano, and a miracle takes place. Without him even being aware of it, his brain has the capacity to sort out all the pieces of the jigsaw and, when asked to play the music again, a month, six months or even a year later, he just sets out the complete puzzle, with no hesitation and so perfectly that it takes a computer transcription to find out any tiny differences there might be from the original.

The problem with these subtleties is that they usually get lost on television producers who want instant and spectacular results. And the production team on the *People* programme was no exception.

Lucy was trying hard to persuade me. Surely he could manage a few bars of something – it wouldn't have to be the whole piece – just so the viewers could get some idea of how he learnt new music?

I should have said 'no' there and then, but a moment's hesitation was all that she needed: 'So, all we need to do is find a piece that will be immediately recognisable to the viewers that Derek's never heard.'

'How on earth are we going to do that?' I scratched my head. 'If most people have heard it, surely Derek will know it too? Really, we ought to choose something obscure, Lucy, or, ideally, get someone to make up a new piece.'

I tentatively offered my services as a composer.

Lucy wasn't having any of it: 'But then the viewers wouldn't be able to tell whether he'd got it right or wrong.'

So I tried to think of music that was well known that I'd never heard Derek play. With some difficulty, I came up with half a dozen possibilities and I fetched him from class to try them out.

With Derek sitting at the piano and Lucy in attendance, I first asked him to play a couple of numbers with which I knew he was familiar to get him warmed up. Then came the new ones.

'And now, how about "The Girl from Ipanema", Derek?' I asked casually. He immediately went into the familiar bossa nova rhythm. Lucy gave me a wry smile. Much the same thing happened with 'When I'm Sixty-Four'. Three songs from shows 'Summertime', 'Oklahoma!' and 'Tonight' from *West Side Story* – followed in the same vein. Lucy's smile was wearing a bit thin. It looked as though the main sequence for her piece on Derek was not going to be possible after all. His repertoire was simply too extensive. There was just one piece left on my hastily scribbled list.

It was important not to let the tension show – Derek was getting wound up enough as it was with all the unusual attention – so I tried to sound as relaxed as possible. 'Thanks, Derek,' I said warmly. 'That was *great*,' as he released his fingers from the final chord of 'Tonight'. 'Now, one last number, please . . . how about 'Memory' from *Cats*?'

But this time he gave no immediate response and so I thought, straight away, that Lucy's problem might at last be solved. It was a curious thing with Derek that he wasn't able to say that he *didn't* know a piece: you had to surmise that this was the case from the fact that he just did nothing instead of starting to play straight away. On this occasion I couldn't afford to get it wrong, though. But how could I check? Usually, to be absolutely sure on occasions like this, I would play him the opening bars of the piece in question, since music was still a far more potent language for him than words, and in any case just because he didn't recognise the title of something wasn't a guarantee that he hadn't heard it before. Most music appeared in his life unannounced on compilation records or tapes.

I drew closer and put my hand on his shoulder. 'Are you sure you don't know it, Derek – "Memory" from *Cats* by Andrew Lloyd-Webber?'

He was silent for a moment, fingers pressed firmly in his eyes, concentrating. The effort it took for him to respond was almost palpable. 'You don't know it,' he repeated quietly.

I looked up at Lucy and nodded.

'That's fine, Derek.' I sometimes wondered if he thought he was in trouble for not knowing a piece. 'No problem. Would you like to learn it?'

'Like to learn it,' he echoed more assertively, sitting up straighter, with a flicker of a smile on his face.

Lucy was looking at her watch anxiously, though. We'd spent so long getting this far that it was now tight for time. 'Do you have a recording here?'

I shook my head.

'Right, we'll have to get it biked over from the BBC.'

An assistant was dispatched to make the necessary arrangements.

Everything was set. The lights were turned on, the cameras were rolling and Lucy gave me the thumbs up to lead Derek into the small hall. She wanted to see him approach the piano as a 'context' shot, apparently. I helped him on to the stool, trying to look natural, and positioned myself on the chair to his right. The *Cats* record still hadn't arrived (we'd heard that the courier had just crossed Hammersmith Bridge) but in the meantime it was decided to get some footage of Derek playing a few of his favourite pieces.

I tried to blank out of my mind the two camera lenses that I knew were staring at us – intent on *not* looking at them, as instructed, which was surprisingly difficult: the urge to give them a sideways glance was almost irresistible. I attempted to ignore the sound man with a fluffy-covered mike on a boom above our heads, tracking our every movement, and I endeavoured not to glance at Lucy and an assistant with a clipboard standing silently behind one of the lights. Just relax, they'd said, you'll be fine.

But I didn't feel at all fine. Despite my best efforts to remain calm, I felt increasingly nervous, and I could sense that Derek was picking up on my unease. One thing I had learnt at music college, though, was how to get through public appearances even when the red mists descended, as one of my teachers put it. Personally, I had never experienced the red mists – instead I had the strange sensation of being frozen, motionless, while at the same time desperately wanting to flee. I could hardly leave Derek sitting there on his own, though, so I took a deep breath and forced myself to speak. 'Right then, Derek, what would you like to play?'

We'd rehearsed our intended verbal exchange several times as we waited to come into the small hall. Since an interview really wasn't on the cards (that was one area where I wouldn't compromise), Lucy was keen to get as much of Derek's speech as she could in a range of everyday situations. At this point he was supposed to respond with '"Don't Cry for Me, Argentina"', so that when Lucy added the voice-over she could explain that this was the first piece I had heard Derek play when he had visited Linden Lodge all those years ago.

Derek just sat silently, however, rocking gently with his fingers pushed up into his eyes as usual.

I tried once more. 'What would you like to play, Derek?'

He sat still for a moment and then almost whispered, 'Like to play?'

One more go, I thought, then we'll have to try something else. 'What would you like to play on the piano, Derek?' I asked one last time, trying to make my voice as cheery and confident as I could.

Again, there was an agonising silence. I gave up. I knew that Lucy wanted him to be seen appearing to decide which piece to perform, but the notion of choice was still a stranger to Derek – even when it had been introduced to him a few moments before.

So I went back to our customary routine: 'Derek, would you like to play "Don't Cry for Me, Argentina"?'

It seemed ridiculous, but those five extra words made all the difference. Freed from having to decide for himself what to do, he immediately sparked into action and, after a brief chordal introduction, the familiar melody got under way. Mentally, I breathed a sigh of relief. But that was only the first part of the problem solved. Lucy had asked us to try managing without two keyboards, preferring to see Derek play on his own. Fair enough, I'd thought, but in the heat of the moment, would he remember to stop?

The indications were not good. Although his playing was rather wooden, the chorus still came round for a third time, and he showed no signs of letting up. I had to stop myself biting my lip. Suddenly it felt uncomfortably hot under the lights. I had to do something, so reaching forward in my chair, I joined him with the tune high up on the keyboard and cued the piece to an end.

A voice said 'cut' and everyone broke into applause as I had asked them to do, so that Derek could get some encouraging feedback on his efforts. I had been worried that, since he would be aware that people were in the room, he might become less motivated to keep trying his best throughout the session if they didn't respond.

Lucy came over to us. 'Well done, Derek,' she said, relieved that after all the discussion and planning they were at last getting some usable material. She indicated to me that she would like a quiet word. 'It doesn't matter if he keeps going on for a bit,' she said gently. 'We'll only be using snippets anyway, so we may as well get a good long take of each piece. Then we'll have plenty of notes to choose from!'

Of course, how stupid of me. As Lucy had said when we first met, since the whole item was only going to be six or seven minutes long and they were going to spend two days filming, the great majority of what was recorded was bound to be discarded in any case.

With that in mind, I started to relax and engage in my customary banter with Derek, so that he too was able to unwind and become more his usual self. As a result, his playing became more expansive in every sense: more notes played with more feeling.

He had just completed his fourth piece, 'The Entertainer', when the single finally arrived from the BBC and there was a short break while the locations of the record player and the lights were checked. Derek and I waited patiently. Finally, all was ready to go and we took up our positions.

I knew what I had to do and on Lucy's cue I came out with the line that I'd mentally been rehearsing for the last few minutes: 'Derek, I want you to listen to a brand-new piece, without playing. And then, when you've heard it, you can have a go. All right?'

'All right, Adam.'

With a reasonably steady hand I set the record going on the turntable (Lucy told me not to worry if it didn't go quite right, since they'd probably want to do close-ups later) and stood while Derek listened intently to the piece – head bowed, engrossed in what he was hearing.

The song came to an end.

'OK, Derek. Your turn.'

And he was off. A little falteringly at first, I thought, but spot on with the tune and the harmonies. He even had a reasonable stab at adapting the arpeggios in the accompaniment to suit his small hands. I was amazed. I really hadn't expected him to do nearly this well. And he just kept going – into the middle section and then back to the reprise of the theme.

Once he'd finished people didn't have to be reminded to applaud: everyone's adulation, including my own, was genuine.

'Derek, that was brilliant!'

'Well done!'

'You really are amazing!'

He just grinned delightedly – clearly very pleased with himself.

I too was delighted but also perplexed. Had the excitement of the occasion somehow swept his mental abilities to new heights? It didn't seem likely, but I didn't have another explanation. As far as Lucy was concerned the answer was simple. She'd been right all along.

We gathered round the television in the drawing room at North Lodge Farm. A number of Derek's family and friends were there, and the boy himself took pride of place, sitting between Nanny and me on the sofa. He could tell that everyone was excited, though I suspected that he had little idea why.

The titles rolled and then Derek Jameson's familiar voice growled across the airwaves.

A 'sh', 'sh' went round the room and the buzz of conversation subsided, to be replaced by a general sipping of drinks as people craned to see the screen.

When he heard Lucy's voice, Derek smiled, and then there he was, playing the piano. Everyone cheered and he clapped his hands in delight. The story unfolded and in due course reached its climax with his feat of 'Memory'. The nation, no doubt, was impressed to hear him doing what for most people was beyond their wildest imaginings. I couldn't resist looking to see people's reactions as he played. Godmother Tisha (as Derek called her) was visibly moved. Mary Ann caught my eye and looked at me quizzically, though she didn't say anything. I wondered what was on her mind.

All too soon, it seemed to the assembled company, Derek's excerpt came to an end. Glasses were recharged and a toast was drunk to Bumpy, the new media star of the family.

Later, when most of the guests had gone and Nanny was putting Derek to bed, Mary Ann and I were left alone in the kitchen. I had to ask: what was it about his performance of 'Memory' that had made her look at me like that?

'It's one of my favourite pieces!' Mary Ann exclaimed. 'Derek must have heard it dozens of times. We call it "Midnight", though.'

I looked at her open-mouthed, shook my head and then we both laughed. I could see now just how false rumours about savant abilities start. We agreed to keep quiet about Derek's unwitting deception for the time being, so as not to spoil things. In any case, there was nothing realistically that we could do, as the programme had now aired. In years to come, though, no matter how many times I tried to put the record straight, the myth persisted. Indeed, despite my unease, the whole sequence was repeated fifteen years later in the BBC documentary *Fragments of Genius* – the programme that also featured Stephen Wiltshire drawing a cityscape of London following a helicopter trip over the capital – and the notion of Derek's instantaneous 'perfect recall' was reinforced. In fairness, *Fragments* did present a more balanced view of his abilities, though, since his extraordinary long-term memory was highlighted too.

All in all, Derek's appearance on the *People* programme was judged to be a great success and the BBC even returned some months after their first visit to film a 'Christmas special' at Linden Lodge – this time featuring him accompanying the other juniors singing carols.

As I looked back, there was no doubt that 1988 had been a good year for Derek and it seemed likely that his appearances on television would represent a peak in his musical activities for the time being. But then, of course, I had no idea of what the next twelve months were to bring.

*

'Right, no cheating!' I scanned the rows of children sitting in front of me in the small hall at Linden Lodge and made sure that all those with any sight had covered their eyes. 'Here we go.'

Leaning over Derek's shoulders I played the first few bars of 'Tie a Yellow Ribbon' in the version I had worked up over the previous months, with which the children were very familiar: using a swing rhythm with chords alternating between the hands. I stopped at the end of the first verse. 'OK, put your hand up if you think it was Derek.'

A number of arms immediately shot up in the air, followed over the next few seconds by some others whose owners were evidently less sure. Meanwhile, a couple of waverers changed their minds and put their hands back down again.

'Keep still and I'll count. 1, 2, 3, 4 . . .'

There were twelve in all, including Derek himself.

'Now, who thinks it was *me* playing?'

Another dozen hands were thrust towards the ceiling – largely, though not entirely, different from the first group.

'Brand, you can't vote twice!' I laughed, reaching over and giving his hand a shake. 'And Derek, you shouldn't be voting at all!' Both of them thought it was funny without really understanding why.

'And last of all, who wasn't sure?'

There were six this time, including Brand and Derek.

'Well guessed, everyone. And the answer is . . .' I hesitated just for a moment to keep them in suspense.

'Derek,' said Derek.

'Actually, it was *me*, Derek.'

'It was *me*,' he echoed.

'No, no, *Adam* was playing – not you.'

'Not you' he returned.

I decided that it was time to get off the merry-go-round before it started on a second cycle. 'Right, no looking again and we'll have round two.'

I tapped Derek on the shoulder and, without either of us needing to say anything, he carried on from where I had left off, matching what he had heard in every detail and producing music that to my ears, at least, was indistinguishable in style from what I'd just played. Some of the children couldn't resist joining in with the chorus – 'Tie a yellow ribbon 'round the old oak tree . . .' – and I let Derek take the music into verse two before gently touching his arm to tell him to stop. Again, no words were necessary. What an enigma he was!

A further show of hands indicated that the children were fairly evenly divided once more. Well, if they couldn't tell us apart, I told myself, then surely no one would be able to. My hunch had been right. At the age of nine, Derek could and did imitate faithfully whatever I did. I was clear in my mind: it was definitely time to find him another teacher.

Not that I had any intention of giving up on my extraordinary young protégé – quite the opposite – if anything, he needed more input, not less. But if he were to grow musically, he would have to absorb influences other than mine, to become immersed in other musical dialects. I envisaged that my role would increasingly become one of co-ordinating the efforts of a number of other teachers over time, managing their interface with him, and all the while encouraging him to develop his own style, his own ideas, his own voice – ultimately, his own musical identity. Back in the early months of 1989 I imagined that this process would take perhaps four or at most five years. In reality, it stretched well into the new millennium.

Finding the right person was never going to be easy. It would have to be a first-rate pianist who could perform in a wide range of styles, including classical, light, pop and jazz; who could play by ear and improvise, and who would be able both to follow what Derek could do and, more important, extend his musical horizons. Clearly, such people did exist at the top of the profession, but was there anyone who would be prepared to make a commitment to teach Derek regularly, to take the time to form a relationship with him, and not be put off by his idiosyncratic behaviour and limited language?

I began the search by asking my old teachers and fellow students at the Royal Academy of Music, but one by one they came back to me without being able to think of anyone suitable. So I put out feelers further afield into the music business, but again drew a blank. Weeks passed and I was beginning to think that the quest was impossible, when Mary Ann got in touch.

She told me that she'd recently had dinner with Zamira Benthall, Yehudi Menuhin's daughter. Zamira had listened intrigued to Mary Ann's account of Derek and the difficulties I had been having in finding a suitable teacher, so she'd given her the name of a contact at the Menuhin School – the specialist centre that the great man himself had set up in the 1960s in Stoke d'Abernon, Surrey.

I duly followed up the lead, more in hope than expectation, since the school had a daunting reputation for educating the very finest young musicians who aspired to careers in the field of classical music. I couldn't imagine that they'd know anyone who'd be prepared to take on Derek.

How wrong I was! The Director of Music listened carefully while I described my talented though eccentric pupil – the wonders and the warts – for there was no point in being anything other than completely truthful. A thoughtful voice sought occasional points of clarification, and then there was a pause. 'Mmm. Let me think.'

For once here was someone who hadn't just said 'no' outright. After a few seconds, I noticed that I was holding my breath. Then the voice came back triumphantly: 'I know – Rachel Franklin. She'd be ideal. She's a wonderful classical pianist, but very good at jazz too.'

I could scarcely believe it. At last . . .

'She's no nonsense, speaks her mind. I think she may get on well with Derek. Her parents run a music club in Denmark Hill. You'll be able to get hold of her through them. I'll phone you back with the details.'

A way forward and what a sense of relief! Perhaps, after all, Derek wasn't destined always to play like me.

*

'Hello, Nanny,' I said cheerily, with Derek skipping along by my side. She was waiting on a bench in the formal gardens at the rear of North House.

'Good *afternoon*, Adam,' she responded warmly. Then, expectantly, 'Good *afternoon*, Bumpy.'

There was a short silence. I squeezed Derek's hand meaningfully.

'Good *afternoon*, Nanny,' he finally piped up and leant forward for the obligatory peck on the cheek.

Val, the school secretary, had phoned me to say that Nanny had been waiting since half past three, though school didn't end until four and I'd told her that we didn't really need to leave until four thirty at the earliest in order to get to Rachel's on time, even with the rush hour traffic. But she'd been happy enough to wait, watching the world of Linden Lodge go by with those eagle eyes of hers. Like Mary Ann, she was a great observer of people – one reason why they had got on so well for so long, I imagined.

'And what have you been doing at school today?' Nanny asked Derek, though I knew that since he would be unable to say what he'd been up to, I was expected to answer.

Hurriedly I tried to recollect what Lina's class did on a Tuesday, though for the most part Derek's life at school charted a similar course irrespective of which day it was: an unobtrusive consistency and routine lay at the heart of Lina's approach. Every morning, when they arrived, the children would take part in 'circle time', during which they took it in turns to greet each other and the three staff, and to find out what was happening that day. Simple as it sounded, this activity could take the five children half an hour or more, as they sought to participate in their own unique ways: sometimes using words, sometimes using sign language specially adapted for blind people, and sometimes using objects that had special meanings. Following the group session there would be individual work using everyday objects and toys, which aimed to introduce and reinforce concepts such as left and right, up and down, same and different – areas of understanding that still largely elude Derek, even today.

As well as these regular activities, each day had its own special event too, helping the children to gain a sense of where they were in the week as it passed by. And thinking about it, I could remember having seen Lina leading the class out to the cluster of shops along the road from Linden Lodge.

'Didn't you go out shopping, Derek?'

'Shopping,' he repeated, rocking forward. As ever, it was impossible to know whether he'd really understood what I'd said and remembered the experience, or whether he was just repeating the word.

The problem was that repetition tended to bring conversation to a halt and I felt obliged to plug the gap: 'Thanks for coming, Nanny. It's good of you to help out.'

Nanny had agreed to act as escort in the car: to keep an eye on Derek and to be around in case of emergencies. She'd clearly come well prepared. I noticed that in addition to her familiar large handbag (which I had learnt over the years contained a full nanny's survival kit, with everything from small change to sticking plasters, safety pins and string), there was also a large, sturdy carrier bag that seemed to be full of provisions of some sort. Folded neatly over one arm was a coat ready for Derek and what looked like a picnic blanket.

'Gosh, Nanny, you didn't carry that lot all the way up the hill, did you?' I asked.

'I may be old but I'm not yet feeble, Adam,' she replied.

'Feeble,' repeated Derek, fancying the sound of the unfamiliar word. 'Feeble, feeble, feeble.'

Time to change the subject, I decided: 'A cup of tea while we wait, Nanny?'

I thought perhaps we could have a drink with the biscuits or crisps or whatever she'd brought with her in the bag. But as we sipped from the sturdy school cups, it remained unopened. I wondered (but didn't like to ask) where she imagined we were going to consume its contents. Perhaps back at school when we returned.

But I was wrong. As soon as we were under way, with Nanny sitting next to Derek in the back of the car, she started setting things out. She spread the picnic blanket across their knees and delved inside the carrier bag. Intrigued, I discreetly adjusted the driving mirror to see what was going on. Nanny pulled out a pack of foil-wrapped sandwiches, a range of snacks, a Tupperware box containing what looked to be slices of fruit and some small drinks cartons of various flavours.

'We couldn't have you going hungry on the way to Rachel's, could we, Bumps? Now, let's start with some *delicious* Marmite sandwiches.'

My curiosity turned to consternation. While I was far from fanatical about the cleanliness of my car (a monthly trip for a wash and vacuum at the local garage was as far as it went), I couldn't imagine what the inside would be like by the time Derek and Nanny had gone thirteen rounds with the contents of the carrier bag.

Catching my eye in the mirror, Nanny paused in the process of feeding Derek small pieces of sandwich. 'Don't worry, I'll clean him up before his lesson.'

'Right,' I answered in a rather strained voice.

'And now, somewhere, Adam, I've got you one or two morsels to keep you going.'

The hand that wasn't engaged in feeding Derek disappeared into the carrier bag again and pulled out a substantial pack of what I assumed to be more sandwiches.

'Oh, thank you, Nanny, you shouldn't have gone to all that trouble,' I gushed, very much wishing she hadn't, but genuinely touched by her kindness. The last thing I felt like doing was eating, while in my mind I was anxiously rehearsing Derek's first lesson with his new teacher. How would he react? How would Rachel respond? I so much wanted things to go well.

I pulled up at one of the numerous sets of lights on the South Circular and carefully opened the package that Nanny had placed on the front seat beside me. There, cut into small, white, crustless triangles, were three rounds of thickly buttered Marmite sandwiches. I put one in my mouth and it slipped down easily enough. Only another eleven to go. But for now I was saved by the change of lights.

Pulling away, I looked back in the mirror and saw that Derek, meantime, was on to his next course. Nanny had opened a packet of crisps and put it on his knees. He could manage snacks like these on his own, but because of his habit of inserting his fingers into every available facial orifice, small flakes of crisp were rapidly getting everywhere, including in his hair and Nanny's, I noticed. I changed gear rather clumsily and the bag and its remaining contents slipped on to the floor.

Nanny tutted and, fumbling behind my seat, managed to rescue some of the crisps. The rest were rapidly scrunched into hundreds of tiny pieces under Derek's restless feet. He enjoyed the sensation and starting stamping gleefully.

'Bumpy, stop that, or Adam will *never* get his car clean.'

I prevented myself from saying something that I might have regretted by filling my mouth with a miniature tower of three claggy Marmite sandwiches. I chewed ruminatively for a few moments, then it dawned on me that all had gone suspiciously quiet in the back of the car. I couldn't resist looking in the mirror once more to find out what was going on. A quick glance revealed that Nanny was dipping once more into her apparently inexhaustible bag of supplies. This time she pulled out a cluster of six pots of fromage frais and a small silver spoon.

No, no, please! But it was too late. Nanny was in full flow: 'Now, Bumpy, would you like Sally Strawberry, Rozzy Raspberry or Andy Apricot?'

'Or Nanny Nut,' I muttered under my breath, for once misjudging the acuteness of Derek's hearing.

He'd heard what I'd said all right, though, and he couldn't resist. 'Nanny Nut,' he said, chuckling and starting to rock.

She was momentarily taken aback. *'I beg your pardon, Derek Paravicini!'* she said very deliberately.

Derek picked up on the warning tone in her voice and sat still for a moment, trying to work out how he might have transgressed. Then he realised what he'd forgotten. 'Nanny Nut, *please*,' he returned, clapping his hands together with a joyous sense of his own mischievousness.

Nanny looked at him with a puzzled frown. Jokes like this were normally planted, in her experience, by Mary Ann. But as there were only the three of us in the car she didn't have to look far to find the source of Derek's wit, and she caught a glimpse of my embarrassed amusement in the mirror. 'And you can pull your horns in too, young man!'

I knew that she didn't really mind, though. We were on the same wavelength as far as Derek's cheeky humour was concerned.

But I could see nothing funny about her efforts to feed Derek fromage frais in the back of the car. The fact that he tended to weave his head from side to side combined with Nanny's lateral angle of attack with a small spoon made it almost impossible for her to hit the target consistently. As I feared, sticky Sally

Strawberry was soon liberally smeared all over the passenger window, door and seat. Derek himself looked as though Nanny had given him a fromage frais face pack. And there were still the drinks to come.

When we eventually arrived at the Crotchets music club we must have looked a truly extraordinary sight. Whatever would Rachel think? As usual, though, Nanny had things under control. Once out of the car, she eased a damp flannel from a small plastic bag and proceeded to wipe Derek down. When it was clear that he was as clean as he was going to get, I rang the bell. Nanny held him firmly by the wrist as he stood on the steps, rocking to and fro in eager anticipation.

We were greeted at the door by a young woman with a fair complexion, brilliant eyes, a broad smile and shoulder-length curls of dark hair. 'You must be Derek. Come in, come in. And Nanny and Adam – hello.'

'Good afternoo . . .' Nanny started to prompt Derek in a stage whisper.

'Good afternoon, Rachel,' he interrupted in a similar tone of voice.

'What's this, a ventriloquist's act?' She laughed.

I flinched, half expecting Nanny to tell Rachel to pull her horns in too, but luckily the jibe seemed to pass her by. In any case, Derek had evidently decided that he liked the sound of this fresh new voice and he instinctively reached out to take Rachel's hand.

She led the three of us into a large, rather subdued front room, which was dominated by a gleaming black grand piano. Beyond that there were a number of upright chairs that seemed to be awaiting an audience. Rachel helped Derek on to the piano stool.

Nanny and I quietly sat down in the front row of the stalls, both wondering (from our different perspectives) what would happen next.

'Well, what would you like to play for me, Derek?' This was the obvious question, of course, but one of the hardest for Derek to deal with.

I was determined not to interrupt, but Nanny had no such scruples: 'What about a nice piece from the Christmas Show, Bumpy?'

For Nanny, the recent school show had been one of the highlights of Derek's career to date, but I cringed inwardly, wishing that the first thing that Rachel heard Derek play could have had a bit more style.

But it was too late, and he set off with 'Christmas in Wonderland' – a song I'd specially composed for the whole school to sing at the conclusion of the entertainment. It was designed to be simple to learn and to have an immediacy that would appeal on first hearing, and Derek added the full range of effects that I'd used on the night, including cascades of church bells at the end. It all sounded strangely incongruous in the hushed atmosphere of the Crotchets music club.

'Well played, Derek,' Rachel said. 'But what on earth was that tat?'

He smiled and I had to laugh out loud. And at that moment I knew that lessons with Rachel were going to work out just fine.

Over the next few weeks she challenged Derek with everything from Debussy and Bartók to Stravinsky and Messiaen, from Fats Waller and Art Tatum to Bill Evans and Herbie Hancock. I could sense his aural palette being extended with a whole new range of colours in sound. For now they remained just that – exotic hues and tints with which he could experiment, that were not yet integrated into his everyday musical vocabulary. Although he knew some of their language, he couldn't yet 'speak' fluently in the tones of Waller, Tatum, Evans, Hancock and the rest. In time, though, I was confident that he would absorb something of their individual jazz dialects into his own improvisations.

Often, Rachel and I would engage in long debriefing sessions on the phone after his Tuesday lessons, discussing what seemed to be working and the areas that Derek was still finding difficult. For me it was marvellous to have an insightful musical mind with which to share the challenge of Derek's extraordinarily convoluted thinking in sound. As the Director of Music at the Menuhin School had predicted, Rachel was just what Derek needed at that time and his musical development took off again.

Every now and then I would come to lessons with specific requests, such as working up a rendition of 'Basin Street Blues' to be performed with a Big Band in Reading just after Easter. On occasions like this the three of us would work out a version with which Derek was comfortable, which he would subsequently use as a basis for his performance at the concert. Rachel would make a tape of what we agreed, and by the following week the music would be there in Derek's mind, his fingers raring to go.

Then, one day late in June, I came to Rachel with a particularly challenging request. I was worried that she would think I was mad and would say so in front of Nanny. I explained that some months before, Mary Ann had been asked to join a committee that was organising the 'Fight for Sight' appeal to rebuild the Institute of Ophthalmology next to Moorfields Eye Hospital. The highlight of the campaign was to be a gala concert – 'Blues to Broadway' – to be held at the Barbican Hall in London. Among the national and international celebrities taking part were the singer-songwriter Peter Skellern, the jazz singer and television personality George Melly with John Chilton's Feetwarmers, and the singer-actresses Bertice Reading and Annabel Leventon. They were to be supported by the Royal Philharmonic Pops Orchestra and the Brighton Festival Chorus, conducted by Neil Richardson.

Given Derek's background, the committee had decided that it would be appropriate to involve him in the concert in some small way and Mary Ann had offered his services in whatever capacity was deemed appropriate: perhaps by playing a short piece at some point in the programme to bring home to people the reason for holding the event.

So far, so good, I could see Rachel thinking – and, as she went on to say, getting Derek to perform briefly (perhaps one of his new Fats Waller pieces?) shouldn't be too difficult.

'But there's more, Rachel,' I confessed.

Having had a quick phone conversation with me and listened to Derek play George Shearing's 'Lullaby of Birdland' down the line, Neil, the conductor, had wondered whether he would like to do rather more than just a short solo. How about a couple of pieces with the orchestra, he had wanted to know. I was so taken aback that, without really thinking through the consequences, I'd just said 'yes'. Derek, I was sure, would love it.

Rachel's expression changed to one of disbelief. She took me to one side. 'Derek's going to play with the Royal Phil? At the Barbican? You must be mad! He's never played with an orchestra before, has he? How's he going to react? He might do anything! He'll probably end up playing all their parts for them.'

I could see Nanny starting to look concerned too.

'It'll be all right, I'm sure. Look, Neil dropped off a tape today of the pieces he'd like Derek to do. All we have to do is get him to play the piano part and it'll be fine.'

I wasn't remotely convinced by my own argument, though, and my stomach was starting to churn.

Rachel said nothing more, but took the tape and put it into the machine by the piano. First up was a straightforward arrangement of 'Call me Irresponsible' for piano and orchestra. Maybe that would be possible. But this was followed by a more demanding version of 'L-O-V-E' by Nat King Cole: there were three verses, each in a different key, with a jazz break in the middle for the piano.

Rachel turned to me. 'When's the concert – some time in the autumn, presumably?'

I swallowed. 'It's on the 18th of July, actually. We've got three weeks.'

I could see her starting to say something, but she changed her mind and instead took Derek's hand and led him to the piano. 'Right, let's get on with it. We've got work to do, Derek.'

Awkwardly, Nanny made her way along the row of occupied seats to join Mary Ann and the rest of the family in the audience at the Barbican Hall. She was flustered, which was not like her at all, and she hated the feeling of not being entirely in control. The final adjustments to Derek's trousers and cummerbund (held up with hidden safety pins at the back) had taken longer than she had expected, and she was afraid of missing the start of the concert. But then the whole of the past three weeks had passed by in something of a whirl.

Extra lessons with Rachel had had to be fitted in. Locating a suitable white silk shirt for a somewhat diminutive nine-year-old had proved far more difficult than she had imagined. Derek's hair had been given a special trim. Meanwhile, the whole of his extended family were getting into a state of high excitement, and the demand for television and radio interviews, and visits from newspaper photographers and journalists had been growing all the time, particularly in the last few days as the publicity for the concert had hit the press.

A nine-year-old blind musical prodigy was to play his first major concert, not just anywhere, but at one of the country's great venues in London, and not just with a local band, but the Royal Philharmonic Pops no less. It was a great story – evidently something very unusual was about to happen – and the media interest had reached fever pitch earlier that day as Derek had arrived for rehearsals at the Barbican. The pressure of the last few hours had been intense and even the stoical, redoubtable Nanny was feeling frayed.

As she made her way to her seat, she smiled briefly at Lina Graham, Brenda Davies, Olga Miller and a cluster of others from Linden Lodge who were sitting a couple of rows further back. Rachel Franklin was there too with an older couple, whom Nanny took to be her parents.

She finally reached her seat next to Mary Ann, who looked pale and anxious, and was fiddling with the programme on her lap. Derek had star billing. Mary Ann couldn't remember ever having felt so nervous in her life. It was one thing having to get through public occasions yourself, but having to watch your children perform was infinitely worse. Was her little boy really about to play in front of these hundreds of people? It just seemed impossible. The formality and professionalism of the players in the orchestra, chatting calming and casually to each other, and sharing the occasional joke as they tuned up, was utterly intimidating.

Then the house lights dimmed, a hush descended and Neil Richardson came on, resplendent in his tails. Mary Ann found herself joining in the ripple of applause that spread across the audience. Neil bowed briefly, turned, raised his baton, and with a flourish took the orchestra into an upbeat opening number.

Mary Ann could scarcely listen. She wondered what Derek was up to now. Was he still in his room or waiting backstage? She could imagine him falling up the steps in his excitement.

All too soon the first piece reached its climax and was received warmly by the full house.

A compère came on, and thanked the audience for coming and supporting the appeal. He paused for a moment and lowered his voice slightly: 'And now, Ladies and Gentlemen, I would like to introduce you to a truly remarkable young man . . .'

Mary Ann gripped her seat. Her face burned in the semi-darkness and her throat was dry.

'. . . playing tonight for the very first time with an orchestra. Ladies and Gentlemen, please welcome Derek Paravicini.'

There was enthusiastic applause. Mary Ann couldn't move, but next to her Nanny was in any case clapping enough for two.

And suddenly there he was, half hidden at first among the violins, fairly skipping across the stage with Adam, who helped him up on to the piano stool. He looked absurdly small and vulnerable sitting there, Mary Ann thought, with the huge grand piano in front of him, his legs dangling over the pedals.

The conductor raised his baton. In the audience, a subdued shuffling and murmuring were hastily squeezed into an expectant silence. Too late, Mary Ann felt the urge to clear her throat.

She couldn't bear to look, but neither could she take her eyes off Derek. She could swear that he was visibly trembling with anticipation, and his fingers were twisting themselves into knots. Neil moved his baton, and there was a quiet chord from the orchestra.

Derek's hands were moving inexorably up towards his eyes. Mary Ann suppressed the impulse to scream.

The orchestra sounded another chord.

She willed him to come in, but the sickening realisation dawned that he hadn't even felt to find where the right notes were.

Agonisingly, Derek slowly started to rock forward.

Mary Ann could no longer bear to look.

In the darkness, time stood still.

There was nothing that she or anyone else could do.

For the first time in his life, Derek was completely on his own.

Nanny, in contrast, couldn't take her eyes off her Bumps. So she had the pleasure of seeing him unlock his fingers at the very last moment and bring his hands down perfectly on the keys for the first chord of 'Call me Irresponsible'. As the notes sounded against the backdrop of the orchestra, Derek's face broke into the broadest, most radiant, beaming smile that she had ever seen. This must be musical heaven for him, she thought.

From his opening chord Derek just took off into the music, weaving elaborate patterns of notes around the orchestra's harmonies that went far beyond the comparatively restrained efforts on the tape from which he had been learning. In an extraordinary moment of emancipation, he freed himself from the shackles of his disabilities and engaged with the orchestra in a mature, witty and above all joyous conversation in sound. Somehow, he imposed *his* will on this most complex of social situations and gripped the audience with his power of musical communication. It was miraculous, unforgettable: one of life's great experiences.

At the end, the applause hit Derek like a clap of thunder and lifted him off his feet. Nanny could see that he was physically shaking with excitement and laughing and applauding himself. She wiped away the suspicion of a tear from her eye. (Nannies don't cry.) Without doubt, this was the proudest moment of her life.

Chapter Six

De Stekels van de Egel

The policeman looked at me suspiciously, though he remained perfectly courteous. 'I see, sir. So you *borrowed* the car to come here today, and now you're not sure how to open the bonnet.'

'Er, yes, that's right,' I replied, feeling rather foolish and fully expecting to be arrested on the spot. The IRA were still a real threat in London and you could hardly get a more high-profile target than the one in whose grounds I was now parked.

'Right sir, if you'd care to give me the keys and step out of your vehicle, we'll see what's what.'

I did as he instructed. As I stood up, I noticed to my relief that Mary Ann, who had lent me her car earlier that afternoon, was standing beside *her* borrowed vehicle further along the row. She seemed to be having similar problems and I called over to her, 'How d'you release the bonnet of your car?'

She explained, then asked in return, 'Any ideas of how to do this one?'

I shook my head. Evidently not all Mercedes bonnet catches were in the same place. You learn something every day, I mused. On reflection, trading up vehicles for the evening hadn't been such a good idea after all.

With the help of a whole posse of policemen Mary Ann's problem was solved eventually. The car was found to be free of explosives and we were able to make our way inside.

With Derek and Nanny in tow we walked up a magnificent staircase to the first floor and were ushered into a reception room at the back of the Palace that overlooked the extensive grounds. A few early comers were sipping cocktails in small clusters around the sides of the room, but my attention was drawn to the grand piano that took pride of place in the centre, its lid open expectantly.

For me, it was always a relief to be able to get on with the music-making with Derek and let others do the social round. So leaving Mary Ann and Nanny to collect their first drinks of the evening, I took his hand and led him over to the fine old Broadwood. 'Shall we get warmed up, Derek?'

We went through some of his usual repertoire while the guests drifted in, although I was saving the best for the formal part of the evening, when our host was due to put in an appearance. I had observed before that it was difficult to keep Derek motivated and playing his best when he was required to fulfil the role of cocktail pianist. Adding to the atmosphere while people chatted over him wasn't his style at all – he liked to be in the limelight and to receive the appropriate recognition for his efforts. So, sitting next to him, I judiciously added a bass-line from time to time as he played, partly to let him know that the two of us were in it together, suffering the ignominy of being ignored, and partly to make him aware that one person at least was listening to what he was doing, so that any deterioration in quality would be noticed.

We were in the middle of the 'Maple Leaf Rag' when I became aware of a hush spreading across the room. Looking up from the keyboard, I saw that Prince Andrew had arrived. Within a few moments Derek's rendition of Scott Joplin's famous piece was the only sound in the room. Drink in hand, Andrew came over to the piano. He indicated that we should keep going and Derek, sensing that people were at last attending to what he was doing, changed down a gear and put his foot on the floor. Where before he had been motoring along in quavers, cascades of semiquavers now filled the room.

'Derek, you are a born show-off,' I thought, although, as ever, I was delighted by his reaction, since without that instinctive sense of occasion – and the ability to rise to meet it – in the future he would never be able to cut the mustard as a mature public performer.

The inevitable applause that followed meant that Derek was itching to go again, but it was Andrew's turn next. He thanked people for coming to the reception at Buckingham Palace and supporting the 'Fight for Sight' appeal, of which he was Patron, and which Derek had so spectacularly helped to kick off at the Barbican two weeks earlier.

We had hardly had time to catch our breath in the intervening fortnight, with a continuous round of recording pieces for television in the UK, the USA and even Australia. There were also interviews and photo calls for a number of papers in Britain including the London *Evening Standard*, the *Daily Telegraph* and the *Sunday Times*, among others. The picture of Derek in his white silk shirt, taken at the last minute in his dressing room at the Barbican, had appeared in newspapers and magazines across the world, in Europe, Africa and Asia.

The media roller-coaster was exciting and alarming at the same time. Just who was in control? (Was anyone?) For good reasons, no doubt, producers and editors had decided that Derek made a good story and the more exposure he got the more was demanded. Journalists competed to search out a new angle on him that would astonish their readers, viewers or listeners even more than the last. While this level of interest could hardly continue, there didn't appear to be an immediate end in sight. Quite by chance, Derek had hit the headlines at a time when there was a general lull in national and international events: memories of the Tiananmen Square massacre in early June were beginning to fade and in London, the *Marchioness* disaster was still three weeks away.

It suddenly registered with me that Prince Andrew was speaking about Derek and I focused again on what he was saying: '. . . a great example to us all. And now I would like to invite him to play for us once again.'

Further applause followed . . . and before I could stop it, the impish thought that had been darting about in my brain for the last few minutes popped out of my mouth. I whispered to Derek what he was to play next and stood back.

He didn't hesitate. A dramatic drum-roll effect on open octaves cut into the last of the polite ovation that had greeted Andrew's speech, then he was off with . . . 'The Grand Old Duke of York'.

There was a moment's silence among the assembled company as people worked out what Derek, with a mischievous grin on his face, was playing. For one awful moment I wondered whether I had badly misjudged the mood of the occasion. But then Andrew burst out laughing as he recognised the piece. There were murmurings from one person to another and soon the whole room got the joke. There was a general chuckling and then applause as Derek brought proceedings to a halt, both up *and* down, with a high chord in the right hand, followed by his trademark 'plonk' on the lowest G that the Broadwood had available.

Among the clapping I could make out certain comments from those who were standing nearest to me.

'Well done, Derek.'

'Fancy thinking of that.'

A woman turned to me: 'There's more to him than you might think.'

She was right, of course, but for the wrong reasons. In any case, whether or not I subsequently came clean, another tale had been added to the corpus of savant folklore.

I caught Mary Ann's eye across the room and winked at her.

She knew what I'd done all right. But she wasn't about to let on either.

Our visual exchange was interrupted as a member of the 'Fight for Sight' committee approached me. He came straight to the point. 'We've got a slot on *Wogan* next week. Would Derek be up for it?'

Having just relaxed, I now felt my heart give an enormous leap. At the time, Terry Wogan dominated the early evening television schedules on the BBC, with three shows a week. These involved him interviewing celebrity figures of the moment in his own inimitable style: relaxed and humorous yet idiosyncratically insightful. To appear on *Wogan* really was the big time as far as the UK was concerned. It would be the natural climax to Derek's current run in the media spotlight and make him a familiar face in millions of households across the country.

But, since the show went out live, it was a highly risky enterprise, equivalent to doing thousands of Barbican concerts all at the same time in terms of the size of the audience that would be reached. All that Derek had done to date paled into insignificance compared with the opportunity – and the potential peril – that now presented itself. It was simply too important a decision for me to take alone on Derek's behalf.

'I'll just have a word with Mrs Paravicini,' I said, and set Derek off with one of his favourite Fats Waller numbers, 'My Very Good Friend the Milkman', which was guaranteed to keep him going for several minutes. Picking up a glass of champagne, I walked over to Mary Ann and Nanny who were deep in conversation with Tisha Monson, who was also on the 'Fight for Sight' committee.

As soon as I could, I politely steered the two of them away from Tisha into a quiet corner of the room and relayed the proposition that had just been made to me.

Nanny had no doubts: she had complete faith in Derek and in my capacity to enable him to deliver. 'Nothing ventured, nothing gained, Adam,' she said. 'What a *wonderful* opportunity!'

I looked questioningly at Mary Ann. Her expression suggested that she was a good deal less certain than Nanny. And had she known then that she would be expected to appear on the show too, her answer might have been different. But as it was, she took what she considered to be the right decision – the only decision – for Derek. 'Go with it,' she said quietly, with the same faith in her son that she had shown ten years earlier when the doctor who had first noticed that he had started breathing had asked her what to do. Derek had succeeded then and she felt sure that he would succeed now.

At two o'clock precisely, the car drew up outside the house in Wimbledon opposite Linden Lodge into which I had recently moved. It had seemed strange leaving my Lutyens-designed room at the school where I had been contentedly ensconced for the previous decade. But I was due to get married in a few days, and 'living in' was no longer going to be practicable. My fiancée Sue and I had met some years earlier when she too was doing voluntary work at Linden Lodge, waiting to take up a place at Corpus Christi College, Oxford to read English. She had herself been a pupil at Linden Lodge some years earlier, before transferring to a grammar school for the blind run by the RNIB in Chorleywood, on the outskirts of London. Before leaving the world of special education, she had decided to put her expertise in Braille to good use and hand down her skills to a new generation of children who were learning to read and write by touch.

As a result of the two of us moving in together, our domestic life was currently in a state of some chaos, with packing cases, an assortment of ill-matching furniture, suitcases with odd collections of clothes, and numerous boxes of books and records piled irregularly in rooms throughout the house. But this disarray was as nothing compared to the scrambled nature of my thoughts: not knowing exactly what was going to happen in the next few hours made it difficult to focus on anything in particular.

As I sat down in the back of the car I pondered again what we had let us ourselves in for. I had learnt that, as Derek was so young (just ten), he couldn't perform live after 7 p.m., so his playing would have to be recorded in the afternoon. Hence that part of the ordeal at least was lessened. The prospect of what was to come was still more than nerve-racking enough though, I mused, as we headed towards Hammersmith, where we were due to pick up Derek, Mary Ann and Nanny from her flat on the way to the BBC Television Centre in White City.

Entering the iconic building for the first time was itself an experience to be relished, though there was no time to dwell on the occasion, as we were whisked away to our dressing room and asked to get Derek ready to perform in half an hour. Nanny soon had him changed and, declining the offer of make-up, we were escorted to a studio where the familiar Wogan set was being assembled.

We were greeted by an efficient-looking man with a clipboard and a headset through which he was constantly giving and receiving information. All around us was an intense bustle of activity as equipment and props were moved into place. Above our heads, racks upon racks of lights were being given last-minute adjustments. I fervently hoped that Derek would play his part well, that all would go smoothly. The pressure was intense, although Derek was oblivious to it. Aware, though, that he would soon be called upon to perform, he was charged up and ready to go.

I longed to introduce Derek to some of the people who were around, so he could at least put names to voices – particularly the man with the clipboard, if he was going to ask him to do things in due course. It only seemed fair to try to explain a little of what was going on, too. But it wasn't going to be easy. Before I could say anything, Mr Clipboard came over and enquired what Derek was going to play.

The producer had asked for something well known and upbeat, and I'd previously settled upon *The Pink Panther* theme, which was instantly recognisable and showed off Derek's technique to the full. It also provided a secure framework on which he could improvise quite effectively, should the mood take him. The production team had made it clear that they wanted Derek to play without me accompanying him on the keyboard, as I yearned to do – however discreetly – to keep things under control. As a compromise, though, they had acceded to my request for a drummer, who would lift Derek's playing, I thought, were he required to do a number of 'takes' and become jaded with no audience to rouse him.

'Does he need to rehearse?' Mr Clipboard asked.

I shook my head, wishing that he would make some effort to engage Derek in conversation. 'No – it's best just to go for it. You'll need to . . .'

But he wasn't listening. 'Positions please!'

Mary Ann and I got Derek comfortable on the piano stool and Nanny gave his hair some final attention before the three of us were bustled out of shot.

Mr Clipboard spoke into his microphone, coloured lights started shining on Derek from somewhere high above, a number of cameramen adjusted their positions around the piano, a voice shouted 'Quiet please', and silence descended surprisingly abruptly.

'Stand by. And . . . *action*!'

I noticed a red light on the camera nearest me flick on, and there, on a small screen, was Derek in profile.

There was a general air of expectation.

Nothing happened.

The seconds ticked by in my head.

Still nothing. Derek continued to rock slowly back and forth on the piano stool.

Mary Ann looked at me, horrified. Nanny shifted awkwardly in her seat. I wanted to shout out to Derek to play.

'Cut!'

Mr Clipboard approached me with an expression of perplexity bordering on exasperation. 'Why isn't he playing anything?'

'No one asked him to. You have to say "Play *The Pink Panther*", then he'll be fine. I did try to tell . . .'

'Right. Let's go again,' he interrupted me.

Once under way, Derek performed creditably enough, though he really warmed up when the drummer joined him. After an animated middle section of which Henry Mancini would have been proud, Derek drove the piece inexorably to its conclusion and threw himself into the final sequence with great panache. His fingers zipped off the last notes in anticipation of the ovation that he knew should follow.

But for the second time in a few minutes nothing happened. Derek rocked slowly on the piano stool, looking puzzled. He knew that there were plenty of people around and that they'd been listening. But why weren't they clapping?

After an age, it seemed, Mr Clipboard said 'Cut' again, and Mary Ann, Nanny and I all shouted 'Well done!' and applauded vigorously, but it was too little too late as far as Derek was concerned. He was now slumped on the piano stool, looking distinctly deflated.

Meanwhile, Mr Clipboard had entered into an intense conversation with someone on the headset. I could guess what was coming – another take – which musically was likely to be as lacklustre as Derek now looked. I had to do something, but Mr Clipboard was already issuing instructions.

'OK, once more. Positions please. Silen . . .'

'Wait!' I cried out, getting up from my seat. 'I need to tell Derek something.'

Mr Clipboard shot me a vexed look. 'As quickly as you can please. We're on a tight schedule.'

Ignoring him, I went over to Derek, whispered something in his ear and gave him a quick hug and a tickle under the guise of adjusting his shirt and getting him to sit up straight. He grinned and reached up to muss my hair, which was a sure sign that he was back in his usual mischievous mode.

I was barely back in my seat when Mr Clipboard was back in the groove: '*Silence*! Stand by. And ... *action*!' Then he remembered his additional instruction. 'Play *The Pink Panther*, Derek.'

This time his performance sparkled from the off with plenty of energy and extra notes.

Mary Ann threw me a questioning look. Whatever had I said to Derek?

I just smiled back with mock innocence, knowing that she'd have to wait for the answer.

'Well?' she asked curiously, when Mr Clipboard had indicated that the second (and thankfully the last) take was complete, and the four of us could return to our dressing room for a while.

'I told him he could give Nanny a good wigging if he played well,' I said just loudly enough so that she and Derek, walking behind us, could hear.

Instantly, both his hands shot up and started rubbing her hair vigorously. It was a family joke that Nanny's full head of hair wasn't all her own, and that if Derek worked at it hard enough, her imaginary wig would come off.

'Well thank you *very much indeed*, Adam,' Nanny retorted, struggling to avoid Derek's strong and agile fingers. 'Stop it, *stop it*, Bumps.'

But by now Derek was laughing too much to care. 'I had my hair done *especially* for today.'

'Sorry, Nanny, all in a good cause – you've got to admit it made him play well.'

Nanny frowned at me, but she couldn't stop her eyes twinkling.

Back in our dressing room, we wondered how we were going to occupy ourselves for the three hours until the show went out. A tight schedule indeed! I needn't have worried about Nanny and Derek, as she had come wisely well-prepared with a bagful of books to read to him, but I could see that Mary Ann, like me, was craving stimulation beyond the four white walls of the dressing room and the adventures of Peter Rabbit.

So we sneaked out for a while into the hot, stale summer air of White City, and she lit a cigarette.

'What did you make of that?'

'A bit too close for comfort. If Derek's going to do much more television, we somehow need to get them to build what happens around him. At least they could have introduced him to the people he was supposed to be working with.'

She nodded, but it wasn't that easy. Back at the BBC, I enquired whether Derek could have a chat with Terry Wogan off air before he interviewed him with Mary Ann and me. That way Derek would be faced with a familiar voice, even if he didn't understand the questions.

My request was noted, but I had a feeling that it would be ignored. The show wasn't run for the convenience of the contributors, and the needs and wishes of the star presenter definitely came first.

After a while I tried again: 'Unless Derek gets a chance to speak to Terry before the show, he won't know who he's talking to and his answers won't make any sense.'

I didn't add that his replies weren't likely to mean much to viewers anyway. At this stage in his life Derek had a repertoire of stock answers to stock questions, most of which concerned everyday events and people at school or at home. Attempt to go beyond these confines and the conversation might as well have been in a foreign language as far as he was concerned. On such occasions, sensing that words of some sort were required to fill the airwaves, Derek would take one of the few options open to him and repeat what he had just heard.

Again my plea was rebuffed, though.

'Don't worry. Terry's a very experienced interviewer. It'll be fine.'

Yes, but I bet he's never interviewed anyone like Derek before, I thought. Having said my piece, however, I felt I could do nothing more. It would be down to Mary Ann and me to manage things as best we could on his behalf as the interview unfolded.

When it finally happened, the whole thing felt every bit as bizarre as I had imagined it would. While Derek's recording was played to the audience, he, Mary Ann and I were somewhat awkwardly positioned on a long piano stool before the self-same instrument. At the time, I couldn't see how the continuity would work, but when I watched a recording later, it did, surprisingly, all seem to make sense.

When the applause had died down, Terry leant over the piano and chatted to Mary Ann and me in his usual nonchalant way.

After two or three questions, Derek decided that he would like a piece of the action too.

'What's your name?' he suddenly blurted out to Terry, to the amusement of the studio audience and, no doubt, millions of viewers at home.

Well, I had warned them. With Derek still so innocent and young – exactly ten years old at the time of the programme – it wasn't a problem. And those watching at home assured us that Derek's piece came across as charming and humorous: touching, even. But it did make me realise just how far we still had to go if he were ever going to mature as a public performer.

For the next few months, Derek was recognised wherever he went. Very often, when he was out and about with family or friends, people would come up to him and chat, and he loved all the attention. People with high voices, low voices, scratchy voices, smooth voices, people with a dog to pat or a child to greet, people with their own story to tell: each interaction helped Derek's social skills advance a little more. And he gradually developed his own menu of simple statements and questions that were enough to get a conversation going:

'Hello.'

'What's your name?'

'How are you?'

'Do you play the piano?'

Answering other people's enquiries of him was always more tricky, of course, because they were unpredictable. What seemed to be obvious questions Derek often found impossible to answer. 'Why do you like music?' and 'What's your favourite piece?' had him stumped. And even 'When did you start to learn the piano?' would produce no response, for the simple reason that he had been much too young to remember. As far as Derek was concerned, there was never a time when he *hadn't* played.

As well as social opportunities, appearing on *Wogan* meant that offers to perform in concerts came thick and fast. For Derek's sake, it was important that we decided how to handle the rush. Derek needed his routine and his education, and I had a full-time job – and a new wife! Between us, we agreed that, as a rule of thumb, we would aim for Derek to take part in one event a month for a while and see how it went. That way, Derek's life wouldn't become too dominated by concerts and he would have plenty of opportunity to extend his repertoire in between times. I had another guiding principle: that, wherever possible, Derek should share the stage with other people. This would mean that he would not always be the centre of attention, and would have the opportunity to listen to other musicians and learn to value their efforts as much as his own.

Even with public appearances restricted to one every four weeks or so, they still seemed to follow each other in quick succession. At the beginning of October 1989, Derek played with the Reading Male Voice Choir in Wargrave, both as accompanist and soloist. At the end of the month he performed with the Dussek Piano Trio in support of the Farm Street Church Appeal in London. There then followed the first in a series of concerts at preparatory and public schools across the country, from Papplewick, Ludgrove and Eton College in Berkshire, to the Dragon School in Oxford and the Downs School in Malvern, and up to Loretto near Edinburgh, as part of a short tour of Scotland. These events were largely initiated through family contacts and, like most of Derek's ventures, invariably became a vehicle to support local, national or even international good causes. Beneficiaries included the MacMillan and Malcolm Sargent Cancer charities, the National Society for the Prevention of Cruelty to Children, Guide Dogs for the Blind, the Royal National Institute of the Blind, the Russian Orphan Support Group, 'Wells for India' . . . the list seemed to be never-ending.

The highlight of Derek's charitable activity around this time, though, was undoubtedly his appearance on the second ITV 'Telethon' in the spring of 1990: a twenty-seven-hour spectacular hosted by Michael Aspel and featuring celebrities from all over the UK. Although the programme was censured by some for what were perceived to be patronising attitudes towards disability, there was nothing remotely tokenistic about Derek's contribution.

As ever, he rose to the occasion, intuitively

building on the experience of the previous twelve months' intensive concertising in a range of venues and with a variety of fellow musicians. In this time I had witnessed him gradually develop as a performer and, while there remained much to do, it was clear to me that he had become technically more robust and musically more reliable. Perhaps most important of all, I sensed that his own voice was slowly beginning to emerge: for while he continued to play pieces in almost every conceivable style, it had become increasingly evident that his musical instincts and strengths lay in ragtime, stride and early jazz. His own natural way of playing sounded more and more like a fusion of popular pianists of the first half of the twentieth century, particularly Scott Joplin, Fats Waller and Art Tatum.

So when we were approached a couple of weeks before the Telethon by the musical director to ascertain what Derek would like to play, Waller's 'Your Feet's Too Big' seemed an obvious choice. There was to be a backing band, which meant that Derek needed to make a tape of his version so that an arrangement could be made and the parts for the other players written out. As it would only be possible to rehearse immediately prior to transmission, it was important that Derek played exactly the same version on the day – at least in terms of overall structure – so the whole thing fitted together. It would be disastrous if, on a whim, he was minded to cut things short or to add an extra repeat of the chorus at the end, for example.

This presented a new challenge with regard to

managing Derek's performance and I decided that an unorthodox approach might work best. I had noticed that as Derek repeatedly played pieces over time, they would progressively evolve as new ideas occurred to him, ideas which would become fixed as features in future renditions. Hence, were he to practise 'Your Feet's Too Big' every day for a fortnight, it might well mutate considerably during that period. Therefore, the safest way of ensuring that the version he had just produced was the one that he came up with live on television was not to have him play the piece in the intervening period; it was better to focus on other things. I judged that it would be prudent to start him thinking about 'Your Feet's Too Big' again in the two or three days leading up to the performance.

The first of the two weeks passed by unremarkably, but at the beginning of the second I developed an ear infection, which quickly laid me low. I decided to confine myself to bed in the hope that a mixture of rest and antibiotics would improve matters speedily. On the contrary, though, both fever and hearing continued to worsen – and just two days before the Telethon I could barely stand. Even more disconcertingly, to the extent that I could hear them at all, pitches sounded slightly different in each ear. There was no way I could see Derek to run through what he had to do, but I hadn't been in touch with him at all for five days, which was unprecedented before a big performance.

Another restless night passed by with no improvement, and with twenty-four hours to go before the programme, I drove the hundred metres or so to my local surgery to request some stronger antibiotics and painkillers. Still I wasn't well enough to spend any time with Derek.

When the next day arrived, I had no choice but to put my emergency plan into operation. I lay in bed, watching my bedside clock until it was 2 p.m. – precisely one hour before the car from the television studios was due. Then I swallowed as many paracetamol tablets as I dared and washed them all down with a large tumbler of water. For one awful moment I thought I was going to be sick, but I managed to hold on while the pills started to take effect. Sweating, I pulled on the necessary jacket and tie, and went downstairs to wait.

As usual on these occasions, Derek had been staying with Nanny in Hammersmith and I smiled weakly at her as they joined me in the car.

Nanny viewed my greyish complexion with horror. 'Are you sure you're going to be all right, Adam?' she asked with real concern.

'I'll be fine, Nanny,' I lied – though it was really Derek I was worried about. In two hours he was due to play 'Your Feet's Too Big' to an early-evening audience of several million people in a version that he had last played two weeks earlier and with a band that he had never heard before. Still, at least we'd be able to have a run-through, I comforted myself, as I lay back and closed my eyes in an effort to stem the feeling of rising nausea.

All too soon, we arrived at the studios and were hurried along to our changing rooms, through to make-up and then to a waiting area just outside the main studio. A number of acts came and went: some dancers, a singer who looked familiar although I couldn't remember her name, and a cluster of newsreaders who were evidently going to do a special routine . . . and then it was Derek's turn.

Rather unsteadily, following the young woman who had been assigned to us, I led Derek into a section of the studio that was in semi-darkness. There was a grand piano, lid open, with a stool for Derek and, a little way back, a chair for me. In the meantime, the studio audience was watching a piece about a beneficiary of the previous Telethon that was being shown on a large screen.

Our escort leant over to me and said something quietly. I gesticulated to indicate that I couldn't hear. She tried again, with exaggerated enunciation, close up to my right ear: 'There's been a last-minute change in schedule, so you're not going to be able to rehearse. You're on after this video. Michael will cue you.'

I started to protest, but what was the point? There was nothing anyone could do now. But it felt like sheer madness. While Derek would no doubt come up with *something* (he always did) there was no guarantee – little likelihood, even – that it would be the version of 'Your Feet's Too Big' that the band were expecting. And who could say how he would react to hearing an unfamiliar accompaniment?

My cogitations were interrupted by a burst of applause that greeted the ending of the pre-recorded piece and, across the studio, attention was focused on Michael Aspel.

My hearing was as bad as ever, my mind was a whirl and I had to use every ounce of concentration to make out what he was saying.

'. . . and now, at the ripe old age of ten, he's here to play "Your Feet's Too Big". Ladies and Gentlemen, Derek Paravicini!'

The lights started to go up on the piano and one caught Derek's face just as he smiled at hearing his name, although I was still in darkness.

It was my one chance to influence things. 'Play it just like the tape, Derek,' I hissed.

And straight away he was off, with the introduction in octaves, exactly as he had done on the tape at school.

Then for Derek there was a magical moment as the band came in, supporting him as he began the main theme. His smile turned to the most enormous grin and, as ever, he took off into the music. His playing was just perfect it seemed to me: fluent and free, yet stylish and controlled; idiosyncratic without being eccentric; exciting without compromising musicality.

I slowly released the breath I had been holding in, but the agony wasn't over yet. It dawned on me that as Derek was enjoying himself so much, he probably wouldn't want to stop. And as I listened, I became more and more convinced that the piece was going on longer than it should. But the lights and cameras seemed to be everywhere, staring at Derek from all angles. I could only move forward to the piano and intervene as a last resort, and it would ruin the effect.

My stomach twisted into a knot. He was approaching another chorus. I made up my mind that if he didn't end it this time then I would act. Again, I found myself holding my breath, listening intently, willing him to wind things up. Please, Derek, end it now. And ... yes, there he went, building up to the climax. Would the band catch on? No ... yes. Brilliant! Great timing together. And suddenly it was all over and the audience were clapping wildly. It was all smiles behind the scenes. Well done, Derek! I shouldn't have worried. He really had moved on since *Wogan* less than twelve months earlier.

What a success! The red illuminated numbers on the giant totaliser above the piano flickered into action as people phoned in with their pledges. It was impossible to say, of course, just how much of the money that was raised that evening was directly attributable to Derek's efforts. But there was no doubt that, in the course of the preceding year, Derek's performances had yielded tens of thousands of pounds for deserving causes, and indirectly, through his ever-loyal family and friends, hundreds of thousands had been raised.

As a result, in recognition of his achievements for others, Derek was later granted the status of a Barnardo's 'Champion Child' – a particularly fitting accolade, since Dr Barnardo was one of his great-grandfathers. Amid much publicity, his award was presented with a number of others at London's

Dorchester Hotel by the Princess of Wales. The ceremony came at an especially turbulent time in her life following her separation from Prince Charles.

As she was introduced to Derek, I wondered whether she was aware that he was a nephew of Camilla Parker-Bowles. I imagined that the peculiar nature of the occasion had not escaped her, though it was hardly a topic of conversation that was appropriate to raise. In any case, there was a sparkle in her eyes and a genuine warmth in her smile as she greeted him – a smile that broadened during the exchange that followed.

Nanny had rehearsed with Derek countless times how to address Her Royal Highness and had repeatedly run through the answers to a number of questions that she had decided Diana would be likely to ask. But in the excitement of the moment, Derek quite forgot his script and, as ever, improvised. 'Hello, Diana, would you like to feel my wart?' he enquired, holding out his hand, on which a small, crusty protuberance had recently erupted.

Stifling laughter, Diana politely declined, but said how much she was looking forward to hearing him play the piano.

'How about "Let's Call the Whole Thing off".'

Nanny shot me a glance, but for once I hadn't prompted him.

She needn't have worried. This time Diana couldn't help laughing aloud. 'Perhaps after lunch,' she said, and then, touching his arm, 'I'll see you later.'

'See you later, Diana, see you later,' replied Derek, smiling and flicking his fingers animatedly, revelling in her engagement with him and sensing that he'd been witty, though without understanding why.

I couldn't help smiling too, though his behaviour, while enchantingly childlike on one level, was increasingly a cause for concern on another. As his musical abilities surged forward, the gap between these and his intellectual and social development was becoming more and more marked. Observing Derek emerge slowly from the shell of childhood, with the turbulent world of adolescence beckoning, it seemed as though he had even further to go compared with his peers who had been interacting with people in age-appropriate ways for over a decade. There was no hiding the fact that in almost every respect Derek was many years behind. Although it didn't seem possible that he would ever catch up completely, the question for me was whether he could somehow convert his delightful childish innocence and charm into something that would be acceptable in an adult. Above all, it was essential that as he physically matured, he would remain someone with whom other people would want to spend time, to engage in conversation, to befriend. If not, then all the patient work that had gone into his music would be in vain and the terrible prospect loomed that he would never be fulfilled.

Looking at him then, as he held my hand tightly, rocking back and forth with excitement and bursting with vitality, it occurred to me that just as I had worked every day for years on helping him to develop his technique to ensure his playing would never be trammelled by technical limitations, now there needed to be a change of focus. As I envisaged his teenage years stretching out ahead of us, it became clear that the same intensity would subsequently be required on supporting the development of his social and communication skills. They had to become the rails on which his music-making would travel rather than the buffers that would prevent its further passage.

I glanced down at Derek again. He was now poking his eyes as his head weaved from side to side and he had started talking to himself; then he broke into laughter – reliving his conversation with Diana, no doubt. Guiding Derek to maturity was a daunting prospect indeed, and perhaps something that would ultimately be impossible to achieve. But I decided there and then that it was a challenge I just had to take up: having come this far with him, there could be no turning back now.

I packed the last of the percussion instruments into a plastic crate and placed it by the door with two others and a keyboard, ready to load up into the car. Since becoming Music Adviser at the RNIB the previous year, many aspects of my life had changed radically. Whereas before my day-to-day existence had necessarily respected the continuities of time and space dictated by the school timetable at Linden Lodge, now I was a free agent, driving up and down the country from my base in West London to support the music education of blind and partially sighted children across the UK.

I hadn't given up everything from my previous way of life, though, and working with Derek still occupied a substantial part of my free time – co-ordinating his piano lessons, organising concerts and taking him out once a week with Nanny to play with a range of different musicians, whose styles of performance and approaches to music-making I hoped he would gradually absorb. All the while, we worked hard with him on developing his repertoire of social skills, suggesting appropriate replies to questions and responses to praise, and practising them over and over again, trying to cajole him out of his echolalia.

For example, when people said 'Well done!' he would invariably come straight back with 'Well done!' himself, which tended to be something of a conversation stopper. So Nanny and I would rehearse commonplace verbal exchanges in the car on the way to lessons and concerts.

'When someone says "Well done!", Derek, you say "Thank you".'

And we would take it in turns to act out what he should say when someone paid him a compliment. He would quickly pick up what to do within the predictable social microcosm of the car, but as soon as he was faced with strangers seeking to make conversation amid the hustle and bustle of real life, all that we had practised seemed to fly out of his head.

'We'll just have to keep working on it, Nanny,' I declared, after a particularly bizarre interchange with a well-meaning member of the public following a concert in Farnham Castle.

'Well played, young man!' a jolly-looking gent had said to the figure oscillating excitedly between Nanny and me.

Unusually, Derek had countered with a question: 'Are you on sleep-in tonight?' Evidently, for some reason residential life at Linden Lodge had popped into his mind.

Surprised but undeterred, the man had persisted, trying to make sense of what Derek had just said. 'I'm sleeping at home,' he'd said thoughtfully. And then, 'Where do you live?'

'Yes,' Derek had responded confidently, 'you do live.' He'd continued rocking for a moment then stopped, clearly thinking about something else. 'The geese.'

Only Nanny and I had appreciated that he'd been referring to the honking guardians of North Lodge Farm, and most people would have given up trying to converse at this point, but the man had demonstrated a certain kindly resolve. 'Is this your grandma?' he'd asked, looking towards Nanny.

Derek hadn't been able to make sense of this question at all, but he'd done his best to offer some sort of reply. 'Your grandma?' he'd echoed. Then he'd had a stab at some names of familiar people. 'Ester?' – and then, as there had been no response, 'Godmother Tisha? Godfather Patrick?'

There'd been another pause, followed by a mischievous smile that suddenly twitched across his face. I'd wondered, with anxious curiosity, what was coming next. 'You must not fiddle with your . . .'

'Thank *you*, Derek,' Nanny had interrupted, for once not concerned to correct his pronouns, the more pressing need being to forestall the hypocorism that she knew was coming. After that, she'd been able to take no more, and even if Derek's social development were to be truncated as a result, she'd brought proceedings to an abrupt end. 'Good evening,' she'd said to the now rather perplexed-looking man. 'We must be getting along.'

But Derek's communication skills were far from my thoughts that Friday afternoon at the RNIB, as I mentally checked that I had everything ready for the music weekend that I was running in the Midlands for visually impaired children and their families. I had hoped to be out of the office shortly after lunch to miss the worst of the rush hour traffic heading out towards the M40. But my plans were potentially compromised by the phone ringing.

I had quickly discovered that people getting in touch was one of the least predictable aspects of my job – there was no way of telling who might be on the other end of the line or what they wanted. It could be an anxious parent making her first contact with a specialist organisation for the blind following her child's recent diagnosis of visual impairment, someone frustrated that his Braille music had not arrived in time for a rehearsal, a government official wishing to discuss a policy issue, or a journalist wanting a comment. So I was in a dilemma: ignore the phone and I might miss something important; but answer it and I might be delayed for a minute or an hour – there was no way of knowing. I hesitated for a moment, but, as ever, curiosity got the better of me, and I walked back over to my desk and picked up the receiver.

A gravelly male voice that I didn't recognise asked to speak to Dr Ockelford. His English was very good, but he was clearly not a native speaker. My initial assessment was that he was German or perhaps Dutch.

'That's me,' I said, sitting down and picking up a pen, for I sensed that this was a conversation that would require notes.

I heard the man drag on a cigarette, before announcing that he was Wim Kayzer, a film director and producer based in Amsterdam. Another inhalation. Was I the right person to speak to in connection with Derek Paravicini, he wanted to know.

Cautiously, trying to imagine what might be coming next, I said yes.

Wim told me that he had seen Derek on television and was keen to involve him in his latest project, a mammoth documentary on memory, to be screened in five four-hour segments.

(He's either a madman or a genius, I thought.)

Wim was bringing together people from across the world: some who were experts on memory, such as Alan Baddeley, and others who, for one reason or another, were exceptional in what they could learn or recall. He particularly wanted the viewers to see Derek in action, listening to a piece and instantly playing it back. Did I think that he would be interested?

Oh dear, here we go again, I thought: the legacy of Derek's performance of 'Memory' all those years ago on the Derek Jameson programme was still casting its long shadow. So I explained how I thought Derek's short-term memory actually worked: that he was not just a tape recorder who could replay exactly what he had heard after listening to it once, but that he initially recreated pieces by recalling salient fragments and features and reassembling them as he played. What he came up with was invariably credible musically. So if a piece were too long or too complicated for him to absorb at one sitting, he would inevitably be inventive when attempting to play it back: reordering the snatches that he could remember, borrowing snippets from pieces with a similar stylistic pedigree or even making up new material if necessary. To me, he perfectly exemplified Oliver Sacks's contention that memory was a form of imagination.

'And it shows that he really is a creative musician, Wim.'

I could sense him listening carefully, drawing periodically on his cigarette. 'So is his memory exceptional, then?' he asked.

'Absolutely,' I replied, 'his *long-term* memory. He must have literally thousands of pieces locked away in his head, all ready to go as soon as you ask for them. He doesn't have to work at it consciously. Mind you, the way his mind works has its downsides too . . .' And I explained that one autistic-like feature of Derek's make-up was that unless you asked him things using the precise form of words with which he was familiar, he was likely to find the request or question incomprehensible. So while his long-term musical memories might well be astonishing in their detail and quantity, getting him to access them could be very difficult.

'It's like . . .' I struggled to find an analogy to explain to Wim what I meant. 'It's like the spines of a hedgehog. Imagine that each memory is a single spine. Touch its tip with precisely the right verbal label and that memory will be open to you. But miss it, even by a tiny amount, and Derek won't have any idea what you're getting at. And he doesn't have the reasoning power to make an educated guess either: he doesn't do "fuzzy logic".'

'Ah,' said Wim, and I could sense him turning the metaphor over in his mind, 'The spines of a hedgehog – *de stekels van de egel*. How interesting. Now, I expect you'd like to hear what I have in mind for the programme. We'll be filming in the "Huis Verwolde", as we call it: an eighteenth-century mansion that started life as a castle in the twelfth century. We're going to have different people in each room.'

He paused for a moment and I imagined him mentally orientating himself in the building, thinking where to start.

'In the library, we're going to have four famous writers talking about what "memory" means to them. Then upstairs, in the turret room, there'll be a man who's lost his long-term memory, and next to him we've got a lady who's in the last stages of Alzheimer's disease. We're going to play her songs from her childhood to see whether any of her musical memories have survived. In the Chinese

Room there'll be three psychoanalysts discussing the subconscious, and I've got some scientists, too. They're going to talk about the different sorts of memories we have, how the brain chooses what to remember and what to forget, how reliable memory is and so on. Elsewhere I'm going to be interviewing people with exceptional memories of one sort or another including, I hope, Derek and Richard Wawro, the savant artist from Scotland.'

Wim told me that he wanted the viewers to have the chance to really get to know the people in the house – and with twenty hours to fill, he would be content for Derek's story to take time to unfold. He would like us to spend a whole day being filmed, playing and talking.

'So, what do you think?' he asked. 'Would Derek like to take part?'

Instinctively, I liked Wim and trusted him, and felt that he would take the trouble to get to know Derek and to put him across in a broadly sympathetic light.

'Pencil him in, Wim,' I said. 'It sounds like quite an adventure!'

I could sense that Nanny's hackles were starting to rise. She glared at the woman across the check-in desk. 'But it *can't* be. I'm sure it's got another year to run.'

Embarrassed, I stepped forward, to see whether I could intervene helpfully: I could detect potential confrontation in the air, since Nanny really wasn't herself. While we'd been waiting in the queue, she'd intimated that it had been a difficult few days at home, with Derek in a volatile and challenging frame of mind – vacillating between appearing withdrawn and anxious, poking his eyes so hard that they were now bloodshot with dark rings round them, and being tense and agitated, rocking frenetically and biting the back of his left hand. For once, apparently, music had provided neither a solace in his fits of depression nor a release of excess energy in his more manic moments. What concerned Nanny even more, though, was the sustained nature of this latest bout of mood swings. Ever since he was a baby, Derek had been inclined to temperamental extremes from time to time, but previously Nanny had always found it possible to restore his equilibrium, through coaxing, distracting or, if necessary, demanding. Now, though, she was finding that the strategies she had relied on in the past with Derek the boy were no longer guaranteed to have the desired effect with Derek the adolescent. Although she would never have admitted it, Nanny felt a weariness that she hadn't experienced before in looking after Derek, and going away to Holland for three days was going to mean digging deep into her reserves of patience and energy.

And now, even before she had managed to check in, there was a problem. Apparently her passport was out of date. But it couldn't be: Nanny prided herself on her attention to detail and she was *never* wrong on issues such as this. The woman at the desk, however, was adamant. 'I'm sorry, Madam, see for yourself. It's two months out of date.' And she handed Nanny the passport.

There was a terrible silence and I saw the colour drain from Nanny's face. For once, she was lost for words.

I felt desperately sorry for her: she was clearly mortified at the prospect of letting people down. All her working life she had set about solving other people's problems, not *causing* them.

I called across to Mary Ann who had been waiting with Derek on the other side of the concourse.

A terse conversation with the woman at the check-in desk followed. There was just an hour before our flight closed and the next sixty minutes were a race against time, as Mary Ann whisked Nanny off elsewhere in the terminal in what surely had to be a vain attempt to obtain a temporary passport.

There was nothing I could do apart from sit with Derek and try to keep him calm. But I was feeling jittery myself and, although he didn't understand what was going on, Derek could sense that something was wrong. His body articulated his unspoken distress as he sat hunched on the chair next to me, fingers and thumbs forced deep into his eyes and mouth, head looping relentlessly from side to side.

The minute hand of the clock on the wall opposite us limped round all too quickly – a quarter of an hour passed, half an hour, three quarters . . . and still no sign of Nanny and Mary Ann.

Like Derek, I felt the irresistible urge to move, and I paced anxiously up and down as he rocked. Ten minutes to go . . . five minutes . . . there had been no other passengers at the check-in for our flight for some time.

Four ... three ... I resigned myself to missing the flight and having to ring Wim to tell him to postpone the filming.

And then suddenly there they were, carving their way through the throng of people at the far end of the concourse, Mary Ann striding ahead, a flushed, distraught-looking Nanny doing her best to keep up.

But in her hand I could see that she was holding a smallish folded card.

'Come on, Derek,' I said, almost yanking his hands away from his face in a sudden release of tension. 'Let's get on the plane.'

But Derek's emotions were trapped in a prison of limited communication and comprehension, and his state of agitation persisted. I began to wonder whether our prospective sojourn in the Netherlands was such a good idea after all.

The Huis Verwolde was every bit as magnificent as Wim had led us to believe and, best of all, as he'd promised, there was a pristine grand piano awaiting Derek in the Chinese room.

Wim suggested that we just 'do what you normally do' for a while and he would film what happened before deciding where to take things next. I acceded gratefully to his request, for I was hoping that Derek would at last be able to relax through a substantial session of music-making and return to something more akin to his usual self. I couldn't wait to get him seated and set him off with some of his favourite Fats Waller pieces, and I wasn't surprised when initially his playing had a frantic, percussive quality – clearly an expression of how he felt.

He crashed his way through 'You've Got Me Under Your Thumb', 'My Very Good Friend the Milkman' and 'Ain't Misbehavin'. I listened patiently, anticipating that things would calm down once the pressure had been released. But to my dismay the opposite seemed to be happening. The more he played the more wound-up he appeared to be getting. Emotionally, he was still locked in his own world and his feelings of frustration were feeding on themselves. I just had to get alongside him musically, to show him that I understood and, if he would allow me, to lead him out of the confines of his mental anguish.

So, with some apprehension, I pulled up a chair to his left and started to add notes in the bass, unobtrusively at first and then more forcefully, stridently – consciously trying to meet him where he was at, and showing him through my playing, in a way that words could never have done, that I appreciated how he felt. Sure enough, he instinctively changed the texture of what he was producing, leaving the bass-line to me and focusing his efforts instead on the upper and inner parts.

Once I sensed that we were united musically, I embarked on the next stage, little by little increasing the intensity of what I was doing, eventually using both hands to create a harsh, jagged accompaniment. Higher and higher discords came to substitute for the original diatonic harmonies and the continuity of the stride bass was deformed through discrete syncopations, contorting the music far beyond the stylistic envelope of early-twentieth-century jazz. But this musical dystopia seemed to encapsulate Derek's feelings more adequately than the symmetries of the original, and his playing too became fractured and dissonant.

In due course, the melody and harmonies of 'Ain't Misbehavin'' were sloughed away completely, leaving only a sequence of naked discords that themselves coalesced into large semitonal clusters that took in each of the twelve available notes, from A up to G sharp. These formed a cacophony that was as clangorous as it was possible to get, and they came to be repeated like hammer blows, louder and louder, and faster and faster – a throwback to Derek's first visceral efforts on the piano when strings were snapped and the mechanism destroyed. But now the force was spread across a clump of notes, and the effect was musically rather than physically destructive.

I glanced across at him. His fingers were being driven at the keys like miniature pistons, the tendons in the backs of his hands were visible like taut steel wires, and his arms were like levers transferring the force from his upper body as he rocked forward to play each chord. The tension was evident in his face, skin tight and lips parted.

On and on the blows rained. Then, just when it seemed as though the storm would never pass, the dynamic level started to reduce, imperceptibly at first, then unequivocally. It was impossible to say which of us started the retreat – maybe we both intuitively felt the urge to pull back from the brink at the same time. Once the process was clearly under way, though, I consciously regulated the change, first through the gradual omission of notes, resolving the semitonal clashes into less jarring whole-tone clusters, and thereafter through a process of gradual transformation into what was technically known as a dominant thirteenth: a chord that signalled the return of the melody. At the same time our playing grew gentler and then more sustained, and by the time we were ready for Fats Waller to return, the music was almost serene. Quieter and quieter our playing became, almost disappearing altogether until, at last, there was the faintest flicker of the tune.

Derek's grimace, which had been softening, was replaced by a smile, which in turn widened into a grin as the tempo picked up again, and both music and pianist returned to their customary jaunty, cheeky selves.

I relaxed and looked around the room. It felt as though we had been away for a while. Two cameras were trained on us and there was Wim, behind them, watching and listening intently.

When 'Ain't Misbehavin'' finally came to an end he came over to us. 'That was excellent, excellent,' he enthused. 'Now, I wonder if I could film you teaching Derek a new piece . . .'

I'd planned on 'Mood Indigo' – strangely appropriate, I thought, in the circumstances.

The rest of the day passed by pleasantly and unexceptionally enough with a good deal of playing and some talking, which was later captured for posterity not only in the documentary but also in a book which Wim produced in Dutch, *Vertrouwd en o zo vreemd* ('Familiar and yet so strange'). Derek appeared to be back to normal: cheerful, co-operative, confident and creative.

As I reflected on the beginning of our session together, it struck me more powerfully than ever before that, for Derek, music wasn't an end in itself, it was the means to an end. The realisation dawned that for him it wasn't just playing the piano that was important, it was making music with and for other people, using it as a vehicle for communication – but he had to be sure that the message was understood and that required interaction with other musicians.

Maybe that's what he'd been missing, I thought, as Nanny, Derek and I were driven back to our hotel that evening. I hadn't been able to spend much time with him of late, and it could be that his other teachers didn't recognise the therapeutic as well as the educational value of music in his life and, thinking about it, they weren't really of that mindset. But neither could I be around all the time to help Derek through his own private *Sturm und Drang* period during his adolescence. Yet if he didn't learn to resolve emotional issues during this time, would he ever be able to? Would he ever make the journey into a mature, balanced and happy adulthood?

I glanced over my shoulder to Nanny, looking tired and drained, who was dozing in the seat behind me and Derek, now as tall as she was, sitting contentedly next to her. For now, for today, all was well as far as he was concerned. But what did the future hold? I could sense the clouds gathering around him, but could see no immediate prospect of shelter from the storm.

Chapter Seven

Loss

'Adam, please, help, can you speak to Mary Ann. She wants a word.'

Nanny sounded distraught – unlike her, always the model of self-control – and straight away I was worried. Had Derek trapped his fingers in a door, I wondered; it was always a possibility that was in the back of my mind. Or perhaps he had been taken seriously ill on account of some long-term consequence of his prematurity of which we had been unaware.

But it was neither of these things. In anxious tones Mary Ann recounted how he had had a 'bad turn', had lost control completely in a fit of rage and frustration. Apparently he had ripped down a pair of curtains in the nursery and thrown a chair across the room, shouting incomprehensibly. He had pulled Nanny's hair and tried to attack her. And he had bitten his own hand so hard that it was bleeding.

My heart sank. This was by far the worst in a series of recent incidents at school and at home that seemed to indicate that the sixteen-year-old Derek was 'going off the rails' as one care worker had put it. What was upsetting him? Who could tell? Despite his rapid physical maturation in the preceding

ADAM OCKELFORD

twelve months, his understanding and language remained in round terms those of a two-and-a-half-year-old, and he couldn't begin to explain what was going on in his head.

Music continued to provide the only release but, as I had discovered in Holland, unless sessions were conceived in what amounted to a therapeutic context, guided by an empathetic musical partner, they were likely to be of little value. Despite repeated efforts, though, I'd had no success in finding anyone who was willing and able to work with him in this way.

In fact, things had recently got worse since his jazz teacher, Peter Muir, who some years previously had taken over from Rachel Franklin on her recommendation, had, like her, gone to seek a new life in the USA. So Derek's specialist musical input was now limited to his 'classical sessions' with Susan Wynn – a visiting piano teacher at Linden Lodge – who confined herself and her pupils strictly to classical fare, in which adherence to the composer's intentions was paramount. While this approach was intrinsically valuable, I sensed that it was not one through which Derek could attain the emotional release that he needed. For him that could only come through the spontaneity of improvisation.

As Mary Ann spoke to me on the phone, my mind was racing. My first instinct was to jump in the car and drive down to North Lodge Farm to see what was going on, but I knew immediately that it wasn't a sensible idea. No matter how upset Derek was, I certainly didn't want him to think that, by throwing furniture around, I (or anyone else) would come running. Equally, though, if he were genuinely distressed (and it sounded as though this was indeed the case), then he deserved sympathy and attention.

'Would you like me to speak to him?' I offered, wondering what tack to take. Should I be firm or gentle? It could be hard to have a conversation with Derek face-to-face at the best of times, and this was over the phone with just the give and take of words, which generally caused him more problems than they solved.

I heard Nanny handing him the receiver, just as a plan of action fell into place in my mind.

'Hi, Derek!' I said, trying to sound positive. 'Mary Ann says you're upset. Can I help?'

There was a pause and then 'Play the piano' came back in response, his voice sounding deeper even than a couple of weeks earlier when we had last conversed. His suggestion suited my hastily conceived strategy well.

'Look, Derek, I'll come and see you at North Lodge tomorrow and we can play the piano then, but you must promise to settle down now and don't throw any more furniture or hurt Nanny. All right?'

Another pause while Derek processed what this offer meant. His cogitations continued for some time.

After a while I prompted him: 'All right, Derek?'

'All right, *Adam*,' he returned with his characteristic articulation, which in recent months had increasingly tended to emphasise people's names.

'Right then, *Derek*,' I responded. 'Have a good night's sleep and I'll see you tomorrow morning.'

'Good night, *Adam.*'

'Good night, Derek. Can you pass me back to Nanny, please.'

He duly handed over the phone.

'I'll come down tomorrow, at about ten, if that's all right with you,' I said. And, aware that Derek would still be picking up what I was saying, 'In the meantime, I told him to settle down and get a good night's sleep.'

Inevitably, the session with Derek the next day was highly charged, and after an hour of running the emotional gamut with him in an extended, tempestuous improvisation in which many of his favourite pieces were woven together and transformed to express his vivid flashes of feeling, I felt drained. When I judged the storm had blown itself out, I left him playing along with a Fats Waller tape and went to join Mary Ann and Nanny in the drawing room.

The discussion that followed was at once open and honest, frank and harrowing. There could be no question that Derek was now in the full throes of adolescence and was evidently being engulfed in wave after wave of inner turmoil. I could only imagine the torment that these uncontrollable surges of emotion were causing him, and the vicarious suffering of Mary Ann and Nanny was almost palpable. Painfully, they admitted to being overwhelmed by a sense of helplessness.

'It must be so frightening for him,' I mused, 'when he gets out of control. I suppose the best we can do when he starts to get agitated like that is to stay with him, tell him that we can see he's upset – that we understand – and that he'll feel better soon.'

'That's all very well, Adam,' Nanny replied, 'but what about if he starts to attack people?' Her voice had an edge to it that I hadn't heard before.

'Move out of range, Nanny, and say that you'll only stay with him if he doesn't hurt you,' I responded quietly.

I could see Nanny wrestling with this notion. It ran contrary to her instincts that any suggestion of weakness in children – the temptation to be misbehave, to be disrespectful, to disobey – should be met by *force majeure*.

Sensing what she was thinking, I tried another angle: 'I don't think Derek's being naughty, Nanny; he really can't help himself at the moment. He's got to work everything through in his own mind – and it's really important that he knows we're going to stand by him, come what may. He needs you now more than ever before.'

And so the conversation moved on. Although it was hard for Mary Ann and Nanny to talk about it, I could tell that the true extent of his learning difficulties was beginning to hit home. While before it had always been possible for them to imagine that he was only a few years behind, and that somehow he would make good most if not all his developmental delay, now, within the space of just a few months, it was plain that the discrepancy between his physical maturation as a teenager and his general level of understanding (akin to that of a preschooler) had become an unbridgeable gulf. The family's hopes and expectations that had been forged during the years of Derek's public acclaim had now become a knife, jagging at an open wound of disillusion.

Other people's attitudes to Derek were changing too. He was no longer the lovable, funny, eccentric little boy, whose faux pas and extraordinary mannerisms were by turns charming and diverting. Overnight, it seemed, Derek the little boy we had grown to know so well had been replaced with a new Derek, a stranger to us all: a young man who for the time being at least seemed to be crushed by his disabilities, whose social gaucheries were embarrassing, even intimidating.

As a consequence – and this was perhaps the hardest thing of all to bear – the requests for Derek to perform had virtually dried up over the last six months or so. The one area where Derek had excelled, the single channel through which he'd been able to reach out into the world of normalcy and wider acceptance, appeared to have been shut off. For sure, he had lost none of the technical precocity that he had developed as a child, but as a young adult, he needed more than that to be accepted as a performer: above all, he needed a distinct and compelling musical voice.

For some time we had been considering Derek's life beyond school. Although he was only sixteen (which meant that he could potentially stay on at Linden Lodge for a further three years), it was important to plan well in advance to ensure that the required funding was in place and, indeed, that suitable provision was available. Here we encountered a major difficulty, since at the time there was nothing in the UK that could adequately meet Derek's virtually unique combination of abilities and needs. The well-established music conservatoires in London and elsewhere that offered the excellence in music education that he required were not equipped to handle his level of intellectual disability, and the colleges that specialised in working with students with learning difficulties did not have the necessary expertise in music.

So with nothing in prospect, I had brought a number of families together, including the Paravicinis, whose sons and daughters were in a similar position to Derek, with a view to setting up a new centre for music and the performing arts intended specifically for visually impaired people with additional needs. As a result, we had established The AMBER Trust – a charity whose initial aim was to raise enough money to get the project under way. Aware of the challenges of going it alone, AMBER had recently entered into partnership with RNIB's Redhill College in Surrey to create what later became known as the Soundscape Centre – a place where Derek and his peers could live out their musical dreams and, wherever possible, awaken equipped to face the demands of the outside world as adult performers.

All this was still some way off, though, as far as Derek was concerned – too long for him to wait, I thought: he needs a significant new musical influence in his life *now* – someone who will help him to find his own voice in music, who will lead him into new stylistic territories, who will expand his capacity for expression through improvisation.

So I wondered aloud with Nanny and Mary Ann whether it would be possible to combine the need for Derek to have a new piano teacher with getting used to life at Redhill College – a more adult environment that might quicken his pace on the road to maturity.

Perhaps I could fix up lessons there once a week, for example.

I agreed to look into it.

It took some time – longer than I had hoped – to find a suitable teacher. I was sure it would have to be a jazzer and someone who was open-minded yet down-to-earth, unfazed either by Derek's extra-ordinary talent or his capricious conduct. I put out feelers into the music community around Redhill and was eventually rewarded with the name and description of someone who appeared to fit the bill. She had been the secretary of a local jazz club, which at the time met at the Watermill pub in Dorking, and she had a reputation for being friendly and unflap-pable, as well as a fine musician. For personal reasons, she hadn't been doing much playing lately. When we spoke on the phone, she admitted that she hadn't done any teaching for a while either. I was curious to know what circumstances had caused her retreat from professional engagements, though I didn't like to pry, and she was in any case happy enough to meet Derek and see how things went.

She was already waiting for us at the college when I arrived with Derek the following Tuesday evening.

'Hi, you must be Ann,' I said, rapidly adjusting my grip to her somewhat diffident handshake. She smiled shyly and nodded. I was struck by her vibrant mass of corkscrew curls, shot through with a range of tints, old and new, that partly occluded a kindly face – a map etched with life's experiences, variously crumpled with humanity and creased with humour. She looked as though she'd only recently woken up. Surely not. But then, she was a jazzer . . .

'And you must be Derek,' she said, turning to him and instinctively touching his arm in greeting.

'Hello, *Ann*,' said Derek. And then, 'You'll play some jazz.'

As part of Derek's recently emerging sense of self, his use of pronouns, which had been static for some time, was at last on the move, and what was conventionally the second person singular now possessed in his terms an exquisite if disconcerting ambiguity: 'you' could mean 'I', 'you' or on some occasions, even more confusingly, both at once.

Ann, of course, took what he said at face value. 'I'm happy to do that, Derek. I hope you'll play some jazz for me too! Now, where're we going?'

As I led the way to the music room, it dawned on me more vividly than ever before that it was through everyday interactions such as this, with people who treated Derek in a matter-of-fact way – just as they found him, just like anyone else – that the key to much of his future development must surely lie. I could see the danger that his social progress would be stunted if he were forever surrounded by people who compensated for his linguistic eccentricities, who constantly made allowances for his intellectual limitations. Hence my primary role should increasingly be not to act as an *intervener* to support Derek's forays into the world of other people (for him an unpredictable and risky enterprise), but to serve as an *interface*: for sure, facilitating and interpreting where required, but not taking all the chance out of encounters, otherwise he would never move on.

The music room was crammed with equipment and instruments that had accumulated pending the completion of the new Soundscape Centre. It was just possible to squeeze by a drum kit and a pair of congas to reach two upright pianos that stood side-by-side against the wall, lids open, beckoning.

I helped Derek find his way to the far piano and then, in accordance with my intention of letting Ann forge her own relationship with him unencumbered by me, I retreated to a chair behind a desk on which stacks of sheet music had been piled.

Avoiding the high hat and snare drum with some difficulty, Ann pushed the stool back from the nearer piano, sat down and swept her hair away from her face.

'So what are you going to play for me?' she asked in a matter-of-fact way, though I imagined that she must have been as curious as I was to know what Derek would come up with.

I was actually more interested to know whether he'd come up with anything at all. Providing an answer to even the simplest of open questions

(Derek, you know *thousands* of pieces!) was still something that invariably eluded him. Whether he lacked the ability, the willingness or the confidence or perhaps a combination of all three, I was still unsure, even after a dozen years of careful observation.

Derek sat rocking slowly on the stool, fiddling with his fingers in his lap. He appeared to be concentrating on Ann's question – perhaps even contemplating a suitable response – though it was hard to judge precisely the point at which his thought processes had become trapped.

The first test of my determination to be an interface rather than an interference was upon me sooner than I had imagined, and for a moment I wished that, like Nanny, I had no qualms about taking control. She would have intervened without compunction at this juncture. But, steeling myself, I managed to keep quiet.

Whatever Ann had been expecting, it certainly wasn't silence.

'Derek, would you like to play me something?' she said quietly, intuitively framing a question that she knew he could answer.

'Yes, Ann.'

'Well, what's it going to be?'

His hands started to move to the keyboard, hovered tantalisingly for a moment, and then retreated once more to his lap. I could see the strain in his face, a flicker of anguish at the failure. That seemingly small step, the short distance in space from his lap to the keys, was simply too great a leap for him to make, intellectually and psychologically.

The agony of it! I started to say something but bit my lip.

Instead I glanced anxiously at Ann, wondering what she was making of her prospective pupil. But she just smiled, a little puzzled perhaps, but apparently calmly accepting of the situation.

'Derek.' Her voice had almost a sing-song quality to it now. (She must surely be an experienced mother, I thought.) 'I've really been looking forward to hearing you play. Now, what's it going to be?'

A short pause and then . . . '"I Got Rhythm".'

My heart leapt and I wanted to shout: 'Well done, Derek!' At last he had achieved this simplest, this most difficult of things. What a breakthrough! Finally he had made a choice for himself without any help from me or Nanny or any other of his puppeteers. Here was evidence that the agonising emotional rebirth of adolescence was at last paying dividends: he had developed enough of a sense of himself to assert *his* will, appropriately, in conversation with a stranger.

He let out a huge grin and this time his hands went straight up to the keys and started to play. (How *did* he know where the notes were without seeming to check first?)

Jauntily, Derek set off with the chorus of the Gershwin classic, tugging at the symmetry of the opening melodic phrase with a series of chromatic harmonies in the left hand and kicking out the rhythmic legs of the middle section with a lively Charleston beat in the right.

Ann leant back on her stool and listened thoughtfully. Derek's playing was becoming livelier all the time, and soon he was fully into his stride, with his preferred leaping bass pattern accompanying rapid flourishes in the right hand.

Then, as sometimes happened, Derek got fixed on one track, and proceedings came to be dominated by somewhat humdrum scales running up and down the top end of the keyboard.

Normally, when this happened, I would metaphorically change the points on his behalf, either verbally or musically nudging him on to a different line of improvisational thought. But I was determined to let Ann take the initiative. How would she react?

I didn't have to wait long. With a trace of a smile she reached forward and started to play an angular line in the right hand, *sotto voce* at first, unobtrusively adding her voice to Derek's soliloquy. After only a few notes, though, he adjusted what he was doing to attend to this novel strand of sound that Ann was now weaving into *his* musical fabric. Almost immediately, the relentless scales came to rest, to be replaced with a series of quiet, detached chords – the weft over and under which Ann passed her colourful new thread with increasing assertion.

Now it was Derek's turn to be intrigued, and before long he couldn't resist trying to emulate what he heard – echoing the jagged line in short energetic bursts. This dialogue gradually evolved into a question and answer routine as Ann left short periods of silence for Derek to fill on his own. After a few minutes, once their explorations appeared to have run their course, she reintroduced Gershwin's famous theme, and the two of them joined forces to bring the duet to a unified close.

As ever, Derek had to have the last word with an extra bass note after Ann had thought things were finished, and then he clapped his hands, delighted and excited by this latest adventure.

Ann's eyes twinkled at his reaction. 'Do you know what that was, Derek?'

'Know what that was?' he threw the question back.

'That was bebop – improvising like Charlie Parker.'

'*Charlie Parker*,' reiterated Derek, relishing the repeated sonority of the vowel sounds.

'Yes – everyone called him "Bird".'

'Bird?' Hearing a familiar word in an unfamiliar context amused Derek. 'Bird!' he said again, and chuckled. Then, evidently playing with verbal associations in his mind, he went on 'Bird, birdie, Birdland ... "Lullaby of Birdland" by George Shearing.'

Triumphantly he realised that through his mental peregrinations he had landed somewhere with a musical resonance and he immediately started to play his fellow Linden Lodger's best-known tune.

I was startled. Two moments of autonomy within ten minutes! At last, connections seemed to be forming between the separate compartments of his mind. At last, those hedgehog spines had decided it was a good idea to do some networking. And best of all, he was starting to network socially too, embarking on his first relationship with a fellow musician unmediated by me. Although I hardly dared to think it, Derek the young adult seemed to be emerging from the troubled chrysalis of adolescence, with a new sense of self and an inner strength and confidence.

Which was just as well, since, unbeknown to us all, Derek was about to suffer the biggest setback of his life.

Looking back, no one (except Nanny herself, of course) was in any doubt that she should have consulted the doctor earlier – though, as Mary Ann reflected when it was all over, there was probably nothing that could have been done in any case. It was entirely in the nature of Nanny's stoicism, though, that she wouldn't let what was – in the early stages, at least – a minor and manageable level of internal discomfort prevent going about life as usual. But deep down, Nanny knew that here was an ache that was something more than an annoying side effect of old age; here was a pain that lay at the very heart of the ageing process itself. And there came a point when she could no longer ignore the gnawing cramps in her abdomen, up under her ribs on the right-hand side, and the heavy feeling of nausea that increasingly assailed her. Unfortunately, by the time of her first consultation with the oncologist, it wasn't just her liver that was implicated and the prognosis was not one of 'whether' but 'when'. Between three and six months, Nanny was told. It was a matter of planning a programme of palliative care.

The family were stunned, dumbfounded, devastated. Everyone had expected Nanny to go on, if not for ever, then at least well into her nineties as her mother had done. All attempted expressions of sorrow and sympathy were brusquely rebuffed by Nanny herself, however. She was robustly fatalistic: her illness and its consequences were God's will and therefore should not be railed against by mere mortals. What was important was to plan practically for the future, particularly, of course, where Derek was concerned.

Despite all her pragmatism, though, it was Nanny's firm desire that Derek should not be made aware of the truth of the situation and, despite profound misgivings, I felt that I had no choice but to respect her wishes. Inevitably, of course, he came to realise that all wasn't well and, indeed, that Nanny was poorly – in itself a new experience for him.

As was the prospect of visiting her in hospital when, a few weeks after seeing the specialist, she was admitted.

Unsurprisingly, there was disagreement as to the best course to take. Some were of the view that it would surely be appropriate to shield Derek from the emotional stresses and strains of seeing someone to whom he was so attached in the intimidating environment of a hospital, with all its sanitary odours and ominously unpredictable sounds. Wasn't there a danger that it would stir some of his earliest, most troublesome, irresolvable memories?

Others felt that since the only place that Derek would be able to be with Nanny before she died would in an unfamiliar healthcare setting, wouldn't it be better for him to get used to it sooner rather than later? Otherwise the shock at the end might be just too much.

Finally it was agreed that I should go with Derek, Mary Ann and Libbet to visit Nanny for a short while to see how things went. If Derek became distressed I could always take him out.

And so it was that on the following Saturday afternoon we duly set off together from North Lodge Farm in Mary Ann's car. It was a hot, bright summer's day and when we arrived at the entrance to the ward the sun was streaming in. All the windows were wide open, and a number of fans were whirring in an effort to keep patients, staff and visitors cool.

I hadn't seen Nanny for some time and I scanned the beds with trepidation, wondering how she would be faring physically as the cancer went about its silent, lethal work. I imagined her looking sallow and gaunt. Distracted by this vision, my gaze was drawn to the second bed on the left, where an elderly lady was lying on her side, unkempt strands of grey hair strewn on the pillow and partly obscuring her face. Clear plastic tubes were taped to her cheeks, which had a ghastly pallor, and disappeared up her nose. Her eyes were closed and there appeared to be no signs of life.

Oh God, surely not. A hot, clammy pulse of fear surged through my body and the room swam. I wanted to run and take Derek, innocently holding on to my arm, with me. He must have sensed my physical reaction and known that something was wrong, because he called out, 'Adam?'

Mary Ann, slightly ahead of me, replied, 'Come on, Bumps!' and she continued to walk further up the ward.

Disconcerted, I peered again at the inert figure lying before me and noticed for the first time a small whiteboard on the wall above the head of the bed. 'Rose Watkins' was scribbled carelessly, barely legibly, in blue felt pen. *It wasn't Nanny*. I shuddered with guilty relief, and turned to follow Libbet and Mary Ann who had now almost reached the end of the ward.

There, partly hidden by a curtain and sitting up in a chair by the bed, was *Nanny*. She was a little pale, but apart from that, looked the same as ever, I thought.

I led Derek up to meet her, swallowing hard in a vain attempt to get rid of the lump in my throat.

She leant forward and reached out to greet him. 'And how's my Bumps?' she asked warmly, looking him up and down. Then she tutted. 'Did no one think to brush your hair before you came out?'

Well, she's not giving up *yet*, I thought. And we started up a stilted conversation about the weather, discussed the assortment of cards – some serious, some droll – that were arranged on a side table and admired the numerous bunches of flowers that occupied a motley selection of vases that were crammed on to every available horizontal surface by her bed.

I struggled unsuccessfully to get Derek to say what he had been doing at home during the summer break. He just sat on the end of Nanny's bed fiddling absently with his hair.

Libbet chipped in, talking about the arrangements for her forthcoming marriage to Bobby Hall.

Mary Ann, always intrigued by life's little details, asked how Nanny was getting on with the hospital food; whether her new medication was making life more comfortable; and what had happened to the good-natured Australian who had been in the bed next to Nanny last time she had visited.

Nanny just gave her a knowing look that somehow managed to make reference to Derek, and the conversation faltered again.

I felt sick and drained, and my face ached with the effort of smiling.

Because whenever I looked at Nanny, the image of Rose Watkins kept floating before my eyes.

Weeks passed by, then months: one . . . two . . . I went to see Nanny whenever I could, usually alone, sometimes with Derek. As I couldn't tell him what was really happening, the visits were even more surreal than they might otherwise have been, with Nanny trying to make it sound as though it was business as usual, as though her stay in hospital was a temporary inconvenience that would soon be over. Deep down, I knew that was exactly what she did feel, though strangely during those last few occasions together we never mentioned her religious beliefs at all. In any case, it was impossible to know what Derek was making of all this and in the end I gave up worrying, taking life as it came, day by day, as Nanny had to.

Then, having been away for a short period I returned home to the phone message from Mary Ann that I had been dreading: Nanny had been admitted to a hospice. It was near North Lodge Farm and visitors were welcome at any time.

She didn't say that the end was near and the tone in her voice was oddly neutral, but I was in no doubt.

I had been thinking about what to do when this penultimate stage was reached. I really wanted Derek to be able to say goodbye in his own way, through the music that he and Nanny had shared all his life.

So, with Mary Ann's agreement, I made the necessary arrangements. I would pick Derek up from home that Sunday evening – complete with his portable keyboard – and we would have a session with Nanny. The receptionist at the hospice confirmed that we could use the communal sitting room and that we wouldn't be disturbing anyone.

It was just getting dark as we arrived, and we were met in the entrance lobby by a nurse, kind and gentle but businesslike in an unobtrusive way, who seemed to know all about Derek already. I shouldn't have been surprised. 'So you're the wonderful pianist that your Nanny's been telling us about,' she said, guiding him to take her arm.

He smiled. 'Yes, the wonderful pianist,' he replied, 'come to play for Nanny.' And he rocked forward in anticipation.

The nurse led us into a fair-sized though otherwise normal enough looking sitting room and asked whether I needed help setting up the keyboard.

I told her not to worry: the coffee table would do well enough as a stand and Derek would be able to reach it by sitting forward on one of the easy chairs.

I had just got everything arranged when Nanny was wheeled in. I had felt strong for the past few hours up until that moment – making the practical arrangements had taken my mind off the reason for us being there. But suddenly the sheer sadness of the occasion was overwhelming and I felt tears welling up in my eyes. I just *had* to be strong, though, for her and for Derek. This was more important than all the concerts we had done put together.

Nanny, a deathly white despite the make-up, but upright as ever, reached up to embrace Derek. 'Now then, Bumps, what are you going to play for me?' The words and the pattern of intonation were Nanny through and through, but the voice was weak and oddly husky. And knowing that her time was limited and keen to get Derek playing, she'd missed out a step in their routine.

Instinctively, Derek filled the gap for her, as she had done for him so many times over the years. 'Hello, Derek,' he said, and then, 'Hello, Nanny.'

After that he was free to answer her question. These days, he could choose at will, and he revelled in trying to select the appropriate piece for the person who had asked him to play. '"Autumn Leaves"?'

More and more, he had the uncanny knack of getting it just right – not only for the person concerned, but for the occasion too.

Spooky, Mary Ann called it.

Despite the inadequacy of the little keyboard and

the physical awkwardness of stretching forward to get at the keys, he played achingly beautifully, or so it seemed to me, with gentle arpeggios adorning the theme, quietly understated, using his fingers to create legato effects in the absence of a pedal.

Perhaps deep down he did understand something of what was happening after all? I just couldn't decide.

Nanny tried to sing along as she had always done, but she was barely able to raise a whisper, feeble now, struggling to wave her arms to the beat.

A medley of her old favourites followed, with Nanny making the supreme effort, but visibly subsiding as Derek carried on oblivious, swaying with the music, thinking that she was still engaged with what he was doing as she had always been.

Despite her frailty, Nanny managed to keep control to the end. 'Last one now, Bumps, then it'll be time for you and Adam to be getting along,' she enunciated in a barely audible tone. And then she ran out of steam, so it was up to Derek to choose again.

With the faintest of smiles playing at the corners of his mouth he pressed down a C major chord and then added a B flat. Almost anything could have followed and, despite the scrambled emotions of the occasion, my curiosity was aroused to know what was coming next.

He started to play a melody, simple and unadorned: a C rising to four Fs and then a snappy rhythm up to A. I recognised it straight away: it was 'Molly Malone'. As the second phrase started, he brought the left hand in, playing the most restrained of harmonies. Here he was reaching back, back in time, to one of his oldest associations with Nanny.

Was it intuition or was it chance?

For Nanny, it didn't matter. She was back in the nursery with him now, a tiny boy with a mop of blond hair rocking to and fro and bashing away at his grandfather's little keyboard. For some reason she was aware too of the sights and sounds of a hot day on Southport beach with Libbet and Derek: she was building sandcastles and he was knocking them over with his little blue plastic spade. It was a glorious summer's day; before them lay a huge expanse of sandy beach, with the Irish Sea in the distance. Now Derek was sitting on the sand in front of her deckchair, losing the unequal battle with his first ice cream. Nanny could feel the warm sun on her back, smell the fronds of drying seaweed and hear the children's voices, laughing and shouting . . .

Derek ended this last piece and waited expectantly for a response. But Nanny's eyes had closed and I was tempted to leave things there. We could quietly make our exit with dignity and Derek would have happy memories of that last session together.

But it wasn't right. He *had* to say goodbye.

'Nanny.' I put my hand on her arm and her eyes opened slightly. 'Nanny, we have to go now.'

This was the part I'd been dreading the most, and I had to bite hard into my lip to make myself carry on. 'Say goodbye to Nanny, Derek,' I muttered to him, knowing that it would be for the last time.

'Goodbye, Nan,' he said, in his usual, matter-of-fact way. And he reached over to give her a kiss.

'Goodbye, Bumps,' she whispered. 'Be good!'

And that was that.

I led Derek out and asked the nurse if he could stay with her for a few moments while I took Nanny back to her room. I wanted to have some time with her alone.

Once there, I sat down on the bed, facing her as she sat in her chair so that we could chat, but she was already drifting away. Her eyes were half closed and there was a period of silence. I was sure she was asleep and was preparing to leave when without warning her eyes opened wide again. 'He won't miss me, you know.'

I was startled, stung. 'Don't say that, Nanny, of course he will, we all will . . .'

The emotion was too much to bear. I could feel my eyes watering once more.

'No he won't . . . he doesn't understand.' There was another pause. 'Anyway it's down to *you* now – you've got to look out for him.'

Suddenly, her eyes came sharply into focus on mine. 'I'm relying on you . . .'

That was the last thing that she ever said to me.

Her head slowly fell forward.

I sat at the end of the bed, not sure what to do. I wiped my eyes. I was too full of emotion to speak. But I had to let her know that I would fulfil her last request.

Could she still hear me?

She was very still.

There was a long pause.

'I'll make sure he's all right, Nanny,' I promised her quietly, taking her hand in mine. 'And I'll make sure he doesn't forget you.'

Chapter Eight

In the Key of Genius

Derek's first term at Redhill College came and went, and that Christmas, at home, everyone commented on how much he seemed to have grown up. He was making more and more choices for himself, increasingly deciding what *he* wanted to do, which pieces *he* wanted to play, and greeting all and sundry with an assertive 'Hi, I'm Derek'.

'I know you are, Derek!' I replied, amused and somewhat taken aback as I greeted him at the front door of his new home in Lambourn – 'the home of the racehorse' – where Mary Ann had recently come to live with her second husband, Toddy Hanbury. After an unsettled decade that had followed her separation and divorce from Nic, it was good to see her more at ease again. And, much to everyone's relief, Derek had taken to his new domestic arrangements with no difficulty.

'How are *you*, Adam?'

'Fine thanks. Get anything nice for Christmas?'

This required more thought, though Derek knew from experience that he was pretty safe in saying 'a CD', since CDs (and, before that, tapes) had been his default gift from most of us for as long as I could remember. More daring experiments from me in the past, a talking watch, for example, had been put away by Nanny for when he was 'old enough to use them'.

But I was determined to break the mould: 'How would you like to come to a musical, Derek, for your Christmas present?'

'Yes please, Adam. *Martin Guerre.*'

I momentarily paused, struggling to keep up with Derek's new assertiveness. *Martin Guerre* had been a favourite of his for some time, ever since he had met Cameron Mackintosh, executive producer of the show. Cameron had played Derek a brand-new number that he had commissioned especially to 'give the opening scene a lift'. To Cameron's astonishment, Derek had been able to play along as he heard the music for the first time. For a moment, Cameron had wondered whether his new number had somehow been leaked – but it was just Derek's amazing speed at processing and reproducing musical sounds that made it seem as though he already knew the piece.

Perhaps more surprising, though, was what happened when Derek met Cameron a year later, as they appeared together at St James's Palace for a charity function. On stage, Cameron introduced Derek to the audience and described how he had first met him. Without further ado, Derek played the song again, this time from memory. However . . .

'I'm afraid *Martin Guerre*'s closed, Derek – so we can't go and see that.'

I wondered how he would react. This was the type of disappointment that could have caused difficulties in the turbulent years of his adolescence.

'What about *Les Mis*, then?'

It was then that I realised that his family was right: Derek really *had* grown up. As she had predicted, Nanny's passing seemed to have had no lasting effects, and his journey towards social and emotional maturity was evidently continuing to follow a slow but steady course.

My mind was racing, though. For a while Derek had been making good progress in his lessons with Ann. She felt that through becoming more familiar with a wide range of jazz styles, his long-held preferences for ragtime and stride had come more clearly into focus – more authentic but at the same time more characteristically 'Derek' – and his playing was more musical, more expressive. However, his career as a public performer had all but been lying fallow for the last two years. This was due in part, no doubt, to the general feeling of inertia that had settled upon us following Nanny's demise, her untiring energy no longer there to charge us up when we started to flag. More important, though, as far as I was concerned, was the fact that it just hadn't seemed appropriate to risk putting Derek before the public's gaze when life had clearly been stressful enough. How would he have reacted, for example, if things hadn't panned out quite as he had anticipated before or during a live performance? Concerts for strangers in unfamiliar venues invariably contained elements of the unexpected.

But now, I sensed, he was ready to start again, doing what he had always loved to do most of all – making music for others.

I made a mental note to contact people in the New Year and let them know that Derek was available again to play for events, large and small. And then, with a new lightness of spirit, I followed Derek into the house to join in with the seasonal festivities.

Gradually, opportunities did come along, and I discussed each with Derek, trying to gauge how he felt. Whereas before, it had seemed appropriate to make most of these decisions on his behalf, since he simply wasn't able to say whether he wanted to take part in a future event or not (although he always seemed to enjoy what was arranged for him), now things had changed. Here was a young man who was fast developing his own views on a wide range of everyday situations. Here was someone who could mentally leap forward into the unknown and imagine, at least in part, what it might be like. Here was a person with an emerging sense of identity, who could assert his own wishes while recognising and increasingly acknowledging those of others. Still, to every offer of a performance he always responded with an enthusiastic 'yes' – though I never took (and would never take) his good-natured willingness to participate for granted.

The first chance to play came in Brecon Cathedral as part of the annual summer jazz festival, courtesy of Derek's father, Nic, who had moved to Wales some years previously with his second wife, Sukie. It sounded like an occasion made for Derek, with a church service that opened to the strains of a Dixieland Band strutting up the aisle playing 'When the Saints Go Marching In', incorporated a number of piano solos, included some stirring hymns and ended with yet more Dixieland jazz. As we had all hoped, Derek revelled in the atmosphere and was keen to continue playing for some time after the service was over.

This success augured well for the future, and next came an appearance at St George's Chapel, Windsor, as part of a year of cultural exchange with Japan. It was a far more formal occasion than Brecon had been, with a classical orchestra supporting a range of soloists. Again, Derek acquitted himself well, supplying lighter interludes of well-known numbers by George Gershwin and Cole Porter in his own piano arrangements.

As Derek's self-belief was re-established, so my confidence in him to deliver the goods grew, and when an invitation to play with Jools Holland, the Rhythm and Blues maestro, came along, it seemed the natural thing to accept. Together, they performed a four-hands set at the Café Royal in London's Regent Street as part of an event to raise funds to equip the Soundscape Centre. I was delighted to see how Derek rose to the occasion through the music – just as he had done when he was little – and by the end of the evening had added a rapid boogie-woogie to his repertoire of bass-lines.

Finally, during this early renaissance period, Derek was offered a spot at Ronnie Scott's, through the good offices of the Beatles producer Sir George Martin – another event that was intended to raise money for Sondscape. This time it was Thelonious Monk who got the Paravicini treatment.

Listening to him jamming along with the house band that Sunday night, I felt that my biggest concern of all was being answered. All through his teenage years, it was evident that for Derek to succeed as a grown-up performer meant that his infant precocity would have to evolve into something more than mere adult eccentricity. He would have to have something worth saying: a distinctive musical voice that was his and his alone; a style of performance that, above all, people would enjoy listening to. Watching strangers' feet tapping along to his rendition of 'Blue Monk' and hearing the spontaneity of the applause that followed, it seemed that the potential was indeed there and was starting to be realised. And most important of all, although he had never been able to verbalise how the trauma of adolescence had affected him and how, in particular, he felt about Nanny's passing, Derek's playing did appear to be getting more expressive than before. Now, it seemed, music was about more than making abstract patterns in sound for which he received the accolade of those around him; it was more than a mechanism for self-release that had helped him through his adolescent years. It seemed that his emotional maturation was matched with the desire and ability to communicate at least some of his feelings *through* music for a wider audience.

I was in no doubt that his career was ready to be relaunched. But how? It seemed unlikely that there would be a repeat of the television exposure that he had had as a youngster – the appearances on high-profile programmes such as *Wogan* that had sparked off such interest across the UK and beyond. How, then, would he be able to reposition himself in people's eyes as a young adult performer?

I suppose I should have anticipated, after so many similar contacts in the past, that the new direction in Derek's life would be determined by a more or less chance phone call from a television researcher. The young woman's voice on the other end of the line informed me that the BBC were considering making a documentary to test out a new theory from an Australian academic – Allan Snyder – that we all have savant-like skills buried within us. He believed that by temporarily 'turning off' some of the higher functioning areas of the brain using powerful electromagnets, subjects would respond to the world around them in purely perceptual terms, uncluttered by the conceptual filtering that prevents most of us from seeing and hearing with the vivid immediacy that (he argued) underpins savant skills.

I listened in silence, wondering if the outcome of the conversation were going to be to ask me for a comment, in which case I was going to have to confess a healthy scepticism. With the musical savants I had encountered, it all seemed to be so much more complicated than that. What about the thousands of hours of practice, for example, that lay at the heart of their special skills? And what was the source of the extraordinary intrinsic motivation that drove their desire to rehearse, hour after hour, day after day, year after year, often in the face of seemingly insuperable cognitive difficulties?

I struggled to refocus on what the researcher was telling me. She had moved on and was talking about recent research in the USA, where it was reported that some patients with degenerative brain disease had quite unexpectedly acquired new skills in drawing and painting that, again, appeared to be savant-like ... (were they really new or had they previously gone unrecognised? I mused) ... and the idea behind the television programme was to bring these two cutting-edge shards of science together to see if the sum added up to more than the parts.

'I don't think either area of research really explains much about the savants I work with,' I confessed, when she had finished, putting my cards on the table straight away in an effort to avoid a protracted discussion where there was hardly likely to be a meeting of minds.

But the researcher's response was disarmingly open: 'I'd be really interested to hear about them. Do you have time?'

I did.

She listened.

And so Derek became involved in *Fragments of Genius*, the first television documentary about savants in the UK since *The Foolish Wise Ones*, made a decade earlier. Along with Darold Treffert's book *Extraordinary People*, the programme had brought the syndrome to public prominence and captured the imagination of many people. The autistic artist Stephen Wiltshire, who had memorably appeared as a young boy in *The Foolish Wise Ones* producing a remarkably accurate pencil sketch of St Pancras station having only seen it for a few moments, was to feature in *Fragments* too. The plan was to have him do something even more spectacular this time – to take a helicopter trip over London and then, immediately on his return to terra firma, to draw the cityscape from memory.

What could Derek do, the producer, Emma Walker, wanted to know, that would have a similar 'wow' factor? I was worried at first in case she wanted Derek to engage in some cheap musical trickery such as playing the piano with his hands the wrong way round on the keyboard, as Mozart had done in the film *Amadeus*. But Emma showed herself to be particularly sensitive to issues around the portrayal of disability and took the trouble to get to know Derek as a person, with several visits to Redhill. For sure, she was blown away by his musicianship, but she was intrigued also to learn what made Derek 'tick', with a view to capturing the essence of his personality on film.

We agreed that there were two main challenges: how to give people an idea of things in everyday life that Derek found difficult without demeaning him, and how to depict his exceptional talents without indulging in freakery. The first problem was solved by showing Derek in what were for him everyday situations – working with an educational psychologist on building up an understanding of numbers and practising his independence skills in the kitchen – but the second issue proved to be more intractable. Unlike the wizardry of Stephen's drawings, which were there for all to see and didn't require an advanced understanding of art to be appreciated, Derek's skills were less tangible. The fact that all the many thousands of pieces in his repertoire were instantly available to him in any key, for example, without any practice (indeed, seemingly without conscious thought or effort) was truly remarkable, but difficult to illustrate in a few moments on screen for a non-specialist audience. And even the speed with which he was able to assimilate new pieces was tricky to demonstrate in a meaningful way for non-musicians. Make what he had to learn simple enough for people to know whether he got it right or wrong and, by definition, the task was going to be very easy. Make what he had to do more challenging and most people wouldn't be able to tell whether Derek had successfully managed the task or not.

Emma took another sip from her drink in the pub where she was drafting the filming schedule following a final 'recce' to see Derek at Redhill. 'So what should we do?' she pondered, toying with her cocktail stirrer.

'Go for sheer virtuosity, I suppose,' I reflected. 'And have him play with a really well-known musician who'll then say what he thinks of his abilities.'

In the event, Jools Holland did the honours and his appearance with Derek had the desired effect of showing him to be a young man who deserved to be taken seriously for his music-making, irrespective of his disabilities. And *Fragments*, which was networked across the USA and, in the years that followed, broadcast in countries all over the world, proved to be the springboard for Derek's life as an adult musician, just as *Wogan* had shot him to fame as a child. Invitations to perform started flowing in once more and, this time, I was determined to establish relationships with concert organisers and fellow musicians that would benefit Derek in the long term.

One of the most intriguing enquiries came from John Lubbock, founder and artistic director of the Orchestra of St John's in London. From its inception at the Royal Academy of Music in the 1960s, the aim of the orchestra was to serve the wider community – seeking to make music accessible to those who might otherwise have had little or no musical experience. And since having his own autistic son, Alexander, John had initiated series of innovative concerts for children with autism and their families. These were musical events of the highest quality which, it was hoped, the youngsters would enjoy and appreciate, but where they could relax and be themselves without fear of censure.

In addition to the light classical repertoire that was performed, John had in the past specially orchestrated arrangements of theme tunes from well-known children's television programmes that were designed to appeal particularly to the younger members of the audience. However, when he heard Derek play on *Fragments of Genius*, he realised that here was someone who could fulfil that function admirably. It seemed that there were no tunes from this recherché repertoire that Derek didn't know, and he played them with such vigour, passion and wit that his arrangements virtually constituted a distinct genre in their own right – something beyond mere pastiche. And hearing *Postman Pat* or *Thomas the Tank Engine* played with such a high level of joyous conviction in the style of Fats Waller or George Shearing had a powerful impact on many of the children. There was something about Derek's playing – an immediacy, an authority that took no prisoners – that seemed to cut through the fault line in perception and understanding that their autism so often produced, and he was able to communicate through music with children who in almost every other situation were locked away in themselves.

The concerts gave Derek the opportunity to work with a wide range of professional musicians too, and he quickly assimilated the typical repertoire of the concerts, playing along with his fellow performers and before long accompanying soloists in classics such as 'The Swan' by Saint-Saëns – a piece with which Derek had been familiar for most of his life. This illustrated another side of his playing that had flowered in young adulthood: his willingness to take a back seat and let others take the limelight.

'Listen and follow what the cello's doing,' I instructed him, as the first rehearsal got under way, and he dutifully paid attention to the tiny changes in tempo that signalled the ends of phrases, and emulated the ebb and flow of the dynamics of the cello – at least to begin with. By the time the main theme came round again, though, he was definitely in the lead and I could sense that the cellist was having to adjust his trajectory to fit in with the big bird on the piano.

'Shhh,' I whispered discreetly in Derek's ear. 'Listen!'

He managed a slight reduction in volume and got back in time with the cello, though it wasn't enough for the boss.

'Quietly!' shouted John testily from the back of the hall. 'And stop playing the cello part. You just do the arpeggios.'

Now, it was an unfortunate quirk of Derek's grasp of musical terminology that he thought the word 'arpeggios' (which are actually broken chords, rather like clock chimes going up and down) meant 'scales' (which are runs involving adjacent notes) and, as ever keen to please, he immediately introduced bold cascades of sound, swirling around the keyboard. The poor swan, which up to that point had been managing to hold its own on what was admittedly an unusually large swell, was now suddenly swamped in sound – musically overwhelmed.

'Stop, stop, *stop*!' John strode up to the stage. 'Derek, what on earth are you doing? It's not supposed to be a storm. You're providing the calm water for the swan to swim on.'

I looked across at Derek anxiously, wondering how he would take to being treated just like anyone else. (John didn't do kid gloves.) But he was absolutely fine, quietly amused at all the fuss and waiting to hear how it *should* be done.

John came across to him and, gently now,

explained what he wanted. 'Like *this*, Derek . . .' and he hummed the rippling introduction. Then, standing behind him, John conducted, using his voice and the occasional physical prompt on the shoulder. '*And* . . . 1, 2, 3, 1, 2, 3, . . .'

Derek concentrated. He responded. Without compromising the intuitive musicality of his playing, he took direction. After a while John stepped back and let him continue on his own.

I too slipped away into the body of the hall to appreciate the interaction between the two musicians more fully; to savour the moment. I had waited so long for this to happen and my heart was lifted still further by the sheer beauty of their playing.

Just as Nannies didn't cry, neither did music teachers get sentimental, but as the swan drifted off into the distance and the piece ended there was a telling silence, and I knew that I wasn't the only one who had been moved.

Then the spell was broken.

'Well done, Derek!'

'Beautiful playing, Derek!'

John slapped him on the back and the other musicians in the orchestra tapped their stands. Just as he had done when he was little, his smile broadened into a beaming grin, and he squeezed his hands together, trembling with excitement.

Derek's reaction was as intense as ever, but there was no doubt that he was in a new place now. His powers of musical communication were beyond question – we had all *felt* them, there in the hall that day; we had each been transported by his playing; and every one of us had had our lives enhanced by his artistry.

Derek had come of age at last.

Coda

I glanced again at the willowy figure on my right, standing half a head taller than me, a hint of a smile playing around the corners of his mouth, his finely sculpted features complemented by a pair of distinctive dark glasses, courtesy of Giorgio Armani.

As he held my arm, I was aware of a regular pattern of tension and relaxation in his body as he swayed slightly from side to side. Occasionally he would rock forward more overtly and flick his free hand so that his fingers snapped together in the air. At the same time, his smile would extend into a grin, and I could feel a pulse of excitement surge through his body.

I thought how comfortable he looked in his black tuxedo and bow tie, white dress shirt, formal trousers and gleaming patent leather shoes: here was a natural performer through and through.

Not for the first time that day, I reflected on the chain of events that had brought us to Las Vegas for the forthcoming concert at the Mandalay Bay Hotel, the climax of our trip to America.

It was over eighteen months since we had first encountered Martin Weitz, who ran a TV production company in Bristol. He had witnessed Derek's extraordinary talents in *Fragments of Genius* and wanted to feature him in a documentary about the brain. But as soon as he saw Derek in action, Martin changed his mind. '*He's* the one I want to make a programme about,' he asserted, as we returned to London from Redhill. 'It may take a while, but I promise you I'll get the backing. He deserves it. What a fantastic young man!'

I smiled and nodded politely, trying not to let my doubts show. On average, I reckoned, about one in five of such projects ever came to fruition, no matter how passionate the proposer seemed on the day. I'd learnt over the years that garnering support for creative ideas was a matter of being both patient and persistent – of keeping several irons in the fire. There was a quiet authority in Martin's tone, though, that made me think that maybe, just maybe, his vision was among the twenty per cent that would succeed. Only time would tell.

During the next year we endured the usual litany of promising leads that blossomed tantalisingly into optimistic plans, before atrophying into regretful rebuffs. Then would follow a period of silence, when I wasn't sure whether Martin had temporarily lost heart in the project or was having no luck in attracting the interest of potential backers.

After a particularly long gap of several months, I came to the conclusion that the venture had run irrevocably into the sand and other possibilities started to bubble back to the surface, among them this biography and a CD. Then, unexpectedly, late in

2005, came the phone call. Martin sounded very pleased and no wonder. A deal had been struck with Channel 5 in the UK and Discovery Health in the USA to put up the funding for an hour's documentary, to be distributed worldwide by Channel 4 International. Derek was to be the main focus of attention, although it would be important to get some additional material from across the Atlantic to satisfy the American audience.

Did I have any ideas, Martin wanted to know.

I said I would think about it. One possibility came to mind, though I couldn't immediately see a way of making it work. My proposal was to do something with Rex Lewis-Clack, a young musical savant who, like Derek, was blind and had learning difficulties. Still only ten years old, Rex too was a pianist with a remarkable ear and prodigious memory. Derek's and Rex's stories had featured in parallel for three years on the *60 Minutes* programme in the segments 'Musically Speaking' and 'Revisiting Rex' thanks to the insights of the producer Shari Finkelstein, who had originally recognised their potential public interest, and Lesley Stahl, veteran CBS correspondent, who fronted the pieces with a genuine warmth and interest. (It was thanks to Derek that Lesley agreed to play the piano on television for the first time, performing a duet with him.) Despite appearing together on *60 Minutes* in the USA, Rex and Derek had never met, however, and the next obvious step seemed to be to introduce them to one another, though a suitable occasion had yet to present itself.

'CBS doesn't make the news, it just reports on it,' Shari told me firmly, when I suggested that she might like to set up a meeting. So it was down to me.

The issue was still in the back of my mind when, a few days after Martin's phone call, an e-mail arrived from Dana Collinson, Events Coordinator for the Lili Claire Foundation, a charity that supports children with neurogenetic conditions, based in California. She had seen Derek on *60 Minutes* and was intrigued to know more about him and the Soundscape Centre at Redhill. She would be coming to London in a couple of weeks; could she pay us a visit?

Everything was duly arranged and Dana listened agog as Derek put her through her paces.

'What would you like me to play for you, Dana?' And when he had finished 'Yesterday' . . . 'Another piece?'

'How about "Somewhere over the Rainbow"?'

He obliged.

Then there was another, and another, and others. Dana couldn't catch him out (few people could, these days) – not that she was trying to. She told us about the large-scale fund-raising events that the Lili Claire Foundation put on in California and Nevada – events that always involved music. 'Would Derek be interested in taking part?'

Something clicked in my mind. Perhaps here was the opportunity I had been waiting for to bring Derek and Rex together.

'Do you fancy going to California, Derek?' I asked.

'*California*,' he reiterated, then off his own bat, 'on a plane?'

'Yes, it would be a long plane journey, Derek. Are you OK with that?'

'OK with *that*!' he said excitedly and clapped his hands.

'That's where Rex Lewis-Clack lives,' I commented, partly to myself, and then explained to Dana what I was hoping to do.

'So, if Rex would like to take part too, and you'd be happy with that, Dana, Martin could arrange for the whole thing to be filmed and he'd have the transatlantic tie-up that he needs. *And* Shari could catch them meeting for the next *60 Minutes* slot.'

Within a week it had all been agreed.

Several months later, and there we were, backstage at the Mandalay Bay Events Center, waiting to perform in the intimidating 12,000-seat arena.

It had been fun meeting up with Rex and his mother Cathleen, though on the whole, rehearsals had been trying affairs. After some debate the artistic director, Keith Resnick, had decided that he wanted Rex and Derek to perform together. It was to be 'The Entertainer', in the style of George Shearing, as Derek liked to do it.

This sounded simple enough in theory, though there were major obstacles to be overcome. Rex was used to making music on his own, and playing with someone else was not on his agenda. So I decided that it would be best to build up to this gradually during the performance by having Rex start on his own and then alternate solos with Derek until they both joined in together at the end with the band. Again, this was fine in principle but, as I soon discovered, Rex was plain unpredictable. With the loyal and tireless Cathleen by his side, though, he could usually be cajoled into playing the right piece at the right time.

In any case I was confident that Derek would carry the day, whatever happened. If Rex did something different on the night, I knew that Derek would be flexible enough to accommodate him. At twenty-six, he was a seasoned performer: reliable, yet bubbling with musical spontaneity and still capable of thrilling audiences with his extraordinary virtuosity.

As he stood next to me now, waiting to go on stage, I was confident that he understood what was about to happen, knew just what was expected of him. He was looking forward to playing with Rex and the other musicians as he had done at rehearsal, and was anticipating the enthusiastic reaction of the audience.

'Where's Ben gone?' asked Derek, as ever interested in those around him, being still for a moment.

'He's with Eric and Kevin, getting some shots of the audience before you play,' I replied.

Derek had become very familiar with the documentary team that had been following us around the UK and across the USA for the last month, and now, with the climax of the whole trip just minutes away, they were like old friends. There was just one chance for Derek and Rex to play and get it right, and one opportunity for them to capture what he did on film and in sound. We were in it together.

Ben Gooder, the director, had surprisingly quickly gleaned real insights into Derek the man and Derek the musician, and was determined to give an account of him that would do justice to his qualities as a fascinating person as well as to his talents on the piano. It was the latter that was principally concerning him now, though, as he came back to join us in the green room with Eric and Kevin, ready to film us walking out and up on to the stage.

'All right, Derek?' Ben enquired. 'All set for "The Entertainer"? There's lots of people out there looking forward to hear you play.'

'All right, *Ben*,' he responded. 'They're looking forward to hearing me.'

He was obviously pleased, and although he looked relaxed and calm enough, I knew that underneath he was excited.

We were interrupted by the inevitable man with a clipboard, telling us it was time go.

'Come on, Derek.'

He was happy to take Ben's arm.

Out in the corridor, Derek's pace quickens as he hears Shari Belafonte singing the Louis Armstrong classic 'What a Wonderful World'. The sound gets louder and louder as we approach the stage. Suddenly, we're there by the steps. Powerfully, professionally, perfectly, Shari and the band drive the music forward to its climax. I see Ben leaning over to Derek and saying something in his ear. Derek acknowledges it and turns round in my direction. I understand. Ben wants Derek to go with me so that he won't be in shot as we go up on to the stage.

As Derek takes my arm, I can feel his visceral reaction to every beat surging through him and out through his fingers like a series of electric shocks. There is no doubt that he is fully charged and ready to go. *His* world is waiting for him on stage.

The music ends. There is cheering and applause. Derek almost physically jumps and he joins in the accolade with a whoop. I can't help laughing.

Eric's camera is trained on us now and Kevin the sound man is with him, keeping an eye on the balance from our radio mics. The compère is starting to introduce Derek and Rex, and I follow what he is saying on the autocue.

It's us! We're on. Derek can't wait to move, but it's best to let Rex and Cathleen go first. Then Derek's reaching for the handrail and up the steps he goes. He's itching to get at the piano, and we stride together across the back of the stage in semi-darkness and then into the spotlights. Derek sits himself down on the piano stool, aware of the audience, waiting eagerly and revelling in the tension of the moment.

I move to the back of the stage again, ready to cue Rex if I have to. The music director looks at me questioningly. I glance at Derek. He is visibly trembling with anticipation, twisting his fingers into knots. I look across to Cathleen and she nods. I give the director a discreet thumbs up.

It's down to Rex now. Will he come in? Cathleen leans over and says something to him. He starts playing. The familiar strains of 'The Entertainer' begin to sound.

But what's happening? He's missed a section.

I look across at Derek. Will he know what to do? As usual, his hands are nowhere near the keys.

The band are unsure what's happening, and if Derek doesn't come in right away and play the missing section, the whole piece is in danger of falling apart.

I watch him intently.

His right hand is reaching up to fiddle with his hair.

I want to scream, but deep down I have faith that he'll come up trumps.

I'm aware that thousands of people and two television crews are wholly oblivious to what is going on, but they won't be for much longer if the music grinds to a halt. The success of the concert and the documentary are now in Derek's hands.

I can't help it: 'Derek!' I shout silently.

But he doesn't need me: he's started to smile and I know that he's sensed what he has to do.

With a flourish, he brings his hands down on the keys and his fingers leap into action.

Derek the musician starts to play.